Em...

New reproductive technologies, such as in vitro fertilisation, have been the subject of intense public discussion and debate worldwide. In addition to difficult ethical, moral, personal and political questions, new techniques of assisted conception also raise novel socio-cultural dilemmas. How are parenthood, kinship and procreation being being redefined in the context of new reproductive technologies? Has reproductive choice become part of consumer culture? *Embodied Progress* offers a perspective on these and other cultural dimensions of assisted conception techniques. Using a multi-sited technique of cultural analysis, this study presents a unique empirical analysis of the experience of assisted conception, whilst also arguing for a 'retooling' of ethnographic method.

Using a range of resources, from media accounts of infertility to parliamentary debate of human fertilisation and embryology, *Embodied Progress* argues for a refashioning of anthropological practice and perspective, as well as a greater understanding of the unique late twentieth-century reproductive dilemmas produced by new forms of choice, technology and scientific progress.

It will be invaluable reading to students and lecturers in anthropology, women's studies and medical sociology and cultural studies.

Sarah Franklin is a Lecturer at Lancaster University.

Embodied Progress

A cultural account of assisted conception

Sarah Franklin

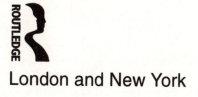

London and New York

First published 1997
by Routledge
11 New Fetter Lane, London EC4P 4EE

Simultaneously published in the USA and Canada
by Routledge
29 West 35th Street, New York, NY 10001

Typeset in Times by
Ponting–Green Publishing Services, Chesham, Bucks
Printed and bound in Great Britain by
TJ Press (Padstow) Ltd, Padstow, Cornwall

British Library Cataloguing in Publication Data
A catalogue record for this book is available from the
British Library

Library of Congress Cataloguing in Publication Data
A catalogue record for this book has been requested

ISBN   0–415–06766–9 (hbk)
ISBN   0–415–06767–7 (pbk)

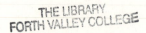

Contents

Acknowledgements

This book had a long gestation, and many people contributed to its formation. I am grateful to Frederique Marglin for introducing me to feminist anthropology at Smith College in 1981. She has been a very distinctive presence in my thinking, teaching and writing ever since. I am also grateful to many of my advisors, teachers and classmates in the graduate anthropology program at New York University, primarily Annette Weiner, Fred Myers, Faye Ginsburg, Hannah Davis and Connie Sutton. It was with the support of a Development Fellowship for two years at NYU that I was able to begin work on the 'virgin birth' debates, much of which was first completed as my MA thesis, and is in part reprinted as Chapter 1. It was also during my graduate training that I was fortunate to meet and to work with Lita Osmundsen, former-President of the Wenner Gren Foundation for Anthropological Research. Her confident encouragement of this research meant a great deal to me and helped make this book possible, as did a dissertation fellowship from the Wenner Gren Foundation in 1987–8. I am additionally grateful to the Wenner Gren Foundation for supporting the 'Politics of Reproduction' Symposium in Brazil, which proved a significant transitional event in placing reproduction centre stage, and which was an enormously valuable intellectual stimulus for all involved. Similarly, Wenner Gren support for an international symposium at the University of California, Santa Cruz, entitled 'What's Blood Got to Do With It? Kinship reconsidered' enabled the beginnings of an equally overdue reinvention of kinship study. This book attempts to contribute to both projects.

I completed the bulk of the research presented here as a doctoral dissertation project at the Centre for Contemporary Cultural Studies at the University of Birmingham, submitted in 1992 under the

Ginsburg-inspired title of 'Contested Conceptions'. The dissertation was supervised by Maureen McNeil, whose intellectual generosity and deep sense of the politics of scholarship continues to be a distinctive source of inspiration. Working with Maureen McNeil, Jackie Stacey and Celia Lury to develop a cultural analysis of Thatcherism in the 1980s greatly clarified some of my thinking around the material presented in Chapter 2, as did my work with the Science and Technology subgroup at CCCS on public debate about reproduction in Britain in the 1980s. I am particularly indebted also to Maureen McNeil for introducing me to the constellation of issues related to science, nature and progress which structures this volume as a whole. *Off-Centre: feminism and cultural studies* (Harper Collins, 1991), which was produced from within the Women Thesis Writer's group at CCCS in the late 1980s, contains much collaborative work that prefigured many of the ideas expressed in *Embodied Progress*.

Outside of my Ph.D. research, I worked as something of a scholar-activist during the 1980s as part of an international network of feminists in several countries concerned with the direction of scientific, legal, medical and ethical developments in the field of assisted reproduction. Across all of the difficult, often disillusioning, lessons of organising to bring about change I was fortunate to work with a number of wise, far-sighted and deeply committed scholars, writers, scientists and health professionals. Among too many people to thank individually are Pat Spallone, Chayanikah Shah, Kamaxi Bhatt, Ferida Sher, Christine Crowe, Lene Koch, Linda Williams, Debbie Steinberg, Annette Burfoot, Vibhuti Patel, Francoise Laborie, Marte Kireczyk, Divya Pandey, Helga Satzinger, Ulla Pensilen, Linda Wilkens, Carme Clavel, Marilyn Crawshaw, Penny Bainbridge, Noe Mendelle, Linda Bullard, Becky Holmes, and Verena Stolcke. The shift away from a simplistic oppositional response to NRTs which informs this book took its inspiration from the unique challenge to feminism of developing critical analytical stances toward techniques such as IVF that are not simultaneously dismissive, demeaning or disrespectful to women who, for reasons this book explores in some depth, seek to 'embody progress'.

Like many of my contemporaries, and previous generations of feminist scholars, I received a great deal of support from the British Sociological Association (BSA), which continues to provide a remarkably open, accessible, and effective network for encouraging research in the social sciences and cultural studies in Britain. In particular, the Human Reproduction Study Group, and the President's Day Associate Section of the British Association for the Advancement of Science on assisted reproduction, organised by Meg Stacey, provided important forums for feedback on the research reported here, and introduced me to a unique group of scholars. In particular, I owe thanks to Margaret Stacey, Naomi Pfeffer, Carole Smart, Frances Price, Erica Haimes, Jim Monach, Hilary Thomas, Hilary Rose, Shirley Prendergast, and Sue Scott.

Shortly after completion of the research for *Embodied Progress*, I was invited by Marilyn Strathern to join her as part of a research team based in the Department of Social Anthropology at the University of Manchester. Funded by the Economic and Social Research Council in 1990, we completed the first multi-sited ethnographic study of 'public' understandings of new reproductive technologies. This work was published in 1993 as *Technologies of Procreation: kinship in the age of assisted conception*, and it was for that project I undertook a detailed, comprehensive analysis of the parliamentary debate of human fertilisation and embryology, which had just been completed as our study began. This collaborative research project provided a unique forum for discussion and debate of specifically anthropological approaches to kinship in the context of new forms of technological assistance to reproduction. My very sincere thanks and appreciations are due to Jeanette Edwards, Eric Hirsch, Frances Price and Marilyn Strathern for the opportunity to benefit from this uniquely stimulating collaborative study.

In 1989, I was also invited to join the Department of Sociology at Lancaster University, where I continue to teach, not far from the birthplace of Louise Brown in Oldham, Lancashire, just down the motorway. I have benefitted greatly from the openness of the Lancaster Sociology Department, in relation to my own work, and through the sheer volume of new work on culture being produced within, or presented to, this department. Work on the 'enterprise culture', globalisation, and 'cultures of nature' at Lancaster has significantly influenced by own understandings of debates concerning technologies, risks, modernities and futures. In addition to ongoing close collaboration with my Lancaster colleagues Jackie Stacey and Celia Lury, I would in particular like to acknowledge the importance of discussions with John Urry, Suzette Heald, Brian Wynne, Russell Keat, Alison Young, Lynne Pearce, and Beverley Skeggs. I was able to complete the final manuscript of *Embodied Progress* with the benefit of sabbatical leave in 1994 provided by the

Lancaster Department of Sociology.

An offer from the European Commission Medical Research Division's Human Genome Initiative, under their Ethical, Legal and Social Implications programme, provided a second opportunity for collaborative anthropological research on kinship and the new genetic technologies based in Manchester in 1992–3. This project, offering a very preliminary analysis of existing anthropological literature on kinship in Europe in terms of its relevance for the understanding of 'implications' related to genome mapping, also significantly shaped my ideas about the continuity of the germline, the history of the ideas of 'life' and of 'genes' in Europe and in Britain, and in particular the historical significance in Europe of the blood-based, bilateral kinship pattern which anticipates the geneticisation of consanguinity. Ongoing discussions with Marilyn Strathern, the Principal Investigator on the EC project, directly influenced the overall models of kinship and gender with which this book engages, as well as the models of conception, procreation and heredity it seeks to interrogate.

Visiting positions at the Department of Anthropology at New York University, and subsequently with the Anthropology Board at the University of California at Santa Cruz, in the academic years 1993–4 and 1994–5 respectively, provided the opportunity to present the penultimate stages of work-in-progress for this book to an American audience. Through my teaching, research and speaking engagements in the United States, I was able to sharpen my sense of what is particularly British, or English, about many of the cultural practices described in this account. The most significant result of my extended stay in the United States while completing this book was a heightened appreciation of the intellectual and political importance of developing new approaches to culture, to methods of cultural analysis, to ethnographic representation, and to specific subject areas such as the study of science as culture. Some of my concern about the tension surrounding issues such as the cultural analysis of science, and the relationship between anthropology and cultural studies, is reflected in *Embodied Progress*, in particular the introduction. I am particularly indebted to Jim Clifford and Sharon Traweek for conversations informing the approaches to disciplinarity, cultural studies, ethnography, fieldwork and anthropology outlined in this book.

Portions of *Embodied Progress* have been presented at numerous conferences, seminars and workshops in North America, Britain,

Europe and elsewhere. In addition to British anthropology departments at Manchester, Keele, Hull, and University College London, portions of this book and arguments from it were presented in the US at Emory University, Stanford University, the University of California San Diego, the CUNY Graduate Center, Yale University, New York University, the University of California Santa Cruz, Rice University, Smith College and UCLA. Of the many colleagues with whom I became newly or re-acquainted in the United States, I would particularly thank a number of readers who provided careful commentary on portions of this book, or papers related to its core arguments: Donna Haraway, Rayna Rapp, Faye Ginsburg, Carole Browner, Cori Hayden, Fred Myers, Annette Weiner, Susan Harding, Helena Ragone, George Marcus, Dorothy Nelkin, Ann Kingsolver and Nancy Chen.

I owe special thanks to students I worked with at New York University, the University of California, and Lancaster University. Much of the important space for dialogue about the burgeoning interest in new reproductive technologies, kinship and conception has occurred in relation to the very exciting research being undertaken by graduate students in the US and the UK. I would in particular like to acknowledge the sustaining, restorative and inspiring input offered at various points by Janelle Taylor, Laury Oaks, Kirsten Dwight, Heather Schell, Cori Hayden, Christine Hine, Stefan Helmreich, Charis Cussins, Cristiana Bastos, Christine Morton, Julian Bleeker and Nick Brown.

Two of the most inspiring people I had the great pleasure of working with, at the very beginning and towards the very end of this project, must be acknowledged in memorium, and I would like here to record a personal acknowledgement to Eleanor Leacock and David Schneider. Annette Weiner, Emily Martin and Carole Delaney must be thanked for putting this book in motion, while Marilyn Strathern, Mary Bouquet and Maureen McNeil gave it much of its shape. Jackie Stacey, Celia Lury and Claudia Casteñeda ensured it reached viability, with help from Wendy Langford, Chris Quinn and Catherine Fletcher. Heather Gibson, my editor at Routledge, commissioned this project and patiently awaited delivery with unfailing optimism, confidence, generosity and a most enabling courtesy. She also proposed Matisse's 1911 'Red Fish' for the cover, which inspiration saw me through the final stretch.

This book is dedicated to the women and couples who very kindly offered to participate in this study, and whose identities must remain anonymous in respect of their privacy. It is their experience for which *Embodied Progress* is entitled, and the dimensions of their experiences which affect us all with which it is concerned.

Sarah Franklin
Lancaster, England

Introduction

This book attempts an anthropological project, though not in the manner accustomed to many anthropologists. The anthropology of contemporary Euro-American societies is becoming more well-established within the discipline, but anthropology retains a strong commitment to its legacy of cross-cultural comparison and its roots in the study of non-western societies. This legacy is, as everyone knows, a contested one, and much has been written on the construction of cultural 'others' within anthropological writings. Hence, contemporary anthropology exists in a state of tension, between the desire to continue to offer ethnographic representations and analysis of cultural diversity, whilst at the same time striving to be conscious of the legacy of its own cultural preoccupations and dispensations in so doing.

Embodied Progress works on the near side of the here and there that defines the anthropological project. By so doing it invites a traffic between the autocritique of anthropological writing and representation, and the continuing project of ethnographic documentation of cultural forms. In this book, the cultural forms are both English and Euro-American, and they are both ethnographically and historically described. This form of description proceeds as a sequence of frames or perspectives. Rather than making all of the connections explicit, the frames are set up to provide room for mutiple refractions.

I begin by revisiting a historical chapter in anthropological theory, namely the celebrated controversy known as the 'virgin birth' debates. I argue in Chapter 1 that these debates demonstrate the importance of a biological model of 'the facts of life' within anthropology. As such, they reveal a great deal about the presuppositions structuring anthropological explanation, not only concerning procreation, kinship and parenthood, but of knowledge, 'truth', empiricism and the effort to be 'scientific'. The givenness of 'natural facts', and in particular the 'facts of life', has allowed them to operate as fixed, unquestionable anchors for much of the history of anthropology, creating for the discipline a particular kind of 'genealogical amnesia' which has only recently been revealed as such (Delaney 1986). The importance of conception to these debates thus has a dual significance: I am concerned both with what anthropologists have had to say about conception, and with their own conceptions of this task. In other words, my focus is on anthropological concepts, as well as anthropological accounts of 'coming into being'.

It is by now well established that anthropology as a discipline cannot claim a purely neutral, objective or value-free approach to the question of cross-cultural comparison, or cultural analysis. Much as anthropology still represents itself as a science in many quarters, the question of what kind of 'science' it can be continues to arouse controversy, often of the visceral variety (Franklin 1995c). While the effort to acknowledge the locatedness of the anthropological enterprise is recognised as an essential antidote to the pretension of offering 'purely factual' descriptions of cultural forms, the precise implications of such a recognition are not agreed-upon. For some, the autocritique of anthropology can 'go too far', resulting in an impoverishment of its capacity to produce useful, reliable, scholarly knowledge. For others, anthropology does not go 'far enough' in widening its project, or allowing a greater diversity of approaches to be incorporated into its own disciplinary reproduction.

Yet, it would be inaccurate to posit, as this phrasing perhaps suggests, that there is some point between 'too far' and 'not far enough' where we might expect a line could be drawn. For it is unlikely ever to be the case that agreement will be reached on this matter. What will occur instead, as is occurring now, is that new kinds of anthropological analysis will be 'born' out of precisely these antipodes. In turn, 'the science question in anthropology' will take on a new aspect. Familiar problems will reassert themselves, past constructions will reappear in a new light, and constructions of the past in turn will alter. As Marilyn Strathern notes, the delightful feature of cultural reproduction is its very reliable tendency never to reproduce itself exactly. And the same can be said of disciplinarity.

Hence, this book is concerned with several levels of reproduction, and disciplinary reproduction is among them. My aim is to contribute to the ongoing reinvention of anthropological theory and method, and by so doing to reinvent its past as well as its future. *Embodied Progress* looks both forward and back. The first chapter looks back at anthropological debates about 'the facts of life', and later chapters look at their contestation in the present and in relation to the future. Whereas the 'natural facts' of human fertility and procreation provided grounds for certainty in the past, contemporary attention to reproductive risk, dysfunction and failure has generated increasing uncertainty. The rapid rise of infertility services in Euro-American societies is the primary context for addressing these uncertainties in *Embodied Progress*. The ethnographic frame is central England in the late 1980s and early 1990s. The central focus is the advent of new reproductive technologies, which are explored from a variety of perspectives. These perspectives, from the popular media, from women who have chosen assisted conception techniques, from public and parliamentary debate of human fertilisation and embryology, and from social theorists who have analysed these different domains, are used as contexts for one another. The aim is to put these perspectives into play, and to develop a perspective on that process.[1]

A perspective is always relational, and relations also have a dual significance in this book. One of the important relations I am concerned with is between the anthropological project and its own past. This has particular significance for my fieldwork, since it was conducted in England, which was home to many of the debates out of which the discipline of anthropology was formed. After many years of living, researching, and teaching in England, I not only read Bronte, Austin and Dickens differently, I read Malinowski, Evans-Pritchard and Radcliffe-Brown differently too. I understood differently the way that Englishness operated in both sets of accounts. This not only gave me a different appreciation of anthropology; it changed how I imagined my own relation to it, which, like being an American in England, has always been slightly uncomfortable, if also rewarding enough to stay longer than I had often thought I might.

It is no coincidence that England is where the world's first test-tube baby was born, in 1978, in Oldham, Lancashire – the same county where I now teach, at Lancaster University (Brown, *et al.*, 1979). England, after all, is the home of a long lineage of scientists concerned with 'the facts of life'. Arguably more than any other country, it has generated enormous scientific interest and accomplishment within the life sciences. From the founding of the Royal Society in London onwards, the modern biological sciences have a special relationship to England.[2] Darwin, Galton, the Huxleys, the Haldanes, Watson and Crick, Steptoe and Edwards, the list is long and by any account distinguished. There are cultural reasons why this is so, and they too have been charted, especially by historians of science, who are also very active on English soil. I discuss these reasons, and the relationship of Englishness to this project, in more depth in Chapter 2.

Englishness also deeply informs the history of anthropology. Although David Schneider claims in his *Critique of the Study of Kinship* that many of the anthropological precepts guiding kinship theory have historically been 'folk models' or 'ethno-epistemologies' of *European* extraction, the description can be more narrowly drawn; they are often explicitly English. Mary Bouquet argues this point both emphatically and persuasively in *Reclaiming English Kinship: Portuguese refractions of British kinship theory* (1993). Specifically, she traces the importance of the notion of pedigree in the formation of the genealogical method by British social anthropologists, which she 'refracts' through her discovery of this model's incommensurability with the kinship universe described by her Portuguese anthropology students. The sense of 'refraction' Bouquet employs to depict the effects of this incommensurability is similar to the model of 'relations' and 'perspectives' I have developed in *Embodied Progress* (see also Bouquet 1996).

The approach taken also affirms the positions argued by Marilyn Strathern in her writings on both English kinship (1992a) and the context of assisted conception (1992b, 1993). It is in Strathern's work that the implications of shifts in perspective brought about by the advent of new reproductive technologies are made visible as a set of cultural effects specific to Euro-American, or English, knowledge practices. Assisted conception thus has a doubled significance in Strathern's rendering: assistance to nature, in the form of what she describes as the 'enterprising up' of kinship, produces consequences in how it is made known. It is the instrumentalisation of the 'facts of life' which makes them differently visible, and thus altered in their significance (their ability to signify). Assistance to conception thus refers both to how conception is technologised, and to its cultural re-conception as a result. This link between reproductive models and cultural knowledge has been formative to the approach taken here.

New reproductive technologies not only create new persons; they create new relations, in both senses of the term. Children born from assisted conception technologies transform a 'couple' into a 'family', for example. The children are themselves 'new relations' in the ordinary kinship sense of relatives, and they also create new relationships: of parenthood and kin connection. The desire to become a family also indexes wider social relations, and the significance of 'becoming a family' in Thatcher's Britain in the late 1980s and early 1990s was distinctive. Thatcher famously claimed that 'there is no such thing as society, there are only individuals and their families'. Her redefinition of British citizenship through the 'enterprise culture' analogy of consumerism had important implications for families and their relatives in England.[3] Couples experiencing infertility often described their disenfranchisement not only from the world of kin and family, but from connections to the wider culture these relations were key to realising. Consumption on behalf of the family, and in particular the option to purchase a family home, were central to the Thatcherite social contract. In the context of an effort to redefine citizenship along the model of 'customers seeking services', the option to purchase costly reproductive services (assisted conception) in pursuit of creating a family, had an overdetermined quality. As one couple I interviewed put it: 'its either a baby or the decorating'. The trade-off, in consumer terms, between procreation and decoration, indexes a particular reproductive model. I discuss the context of Thatcher's Britain, and its relevance to this account, along with other aspects of Englishness, in Chapter 2.

The relative benefits of the baby or the decorating signal the most important reference for this study as a whole, which is kinship theory. Though I am arguing for an appreciation of the artefactual significance of kinship theory in this book, I am by no means arguing for its relegation to the dustbin. I am instead arguing for a specific means of reinventing it, and applying it, as Chapters 3, 4, and 5 make clear. These chapters present the findings of a study of women's experience of in vitro fertilisation, the most important, invasive and 'high tech' of the 'assisted conception' options. This study combined extensive observations in an infertility clinic with in-depth interviews. Twenty-two women, some with their partners and some without, participated in the interview component of the study, and provided accounts of the procedure. These accounts were transcribed, analysed and sorted into themes, which structure their presentation in the second half of the book.

In these chapters I am concerned with several aspects of the relativity that might be described as kinship. Specifically, I have sought to foreground the difference it makes to add technological enablement into the production of new relations. I argue that new procreative technologies not only have implications for definitions of relatedness in the traditional kinship sense of ties established through reproduction. They also add a significant set of new relationships into the kinship equation, and these are the relationships to science and technology. These relationships are quite complex: they are at times tentative, at other times overwhelming, and often confusing. The process of making sense of both new and missed conceptions is productive of new conception stories, and these are the site of much personal, public and parliamentary contestation.[4]

The main refraction organising this book thus becomes apparent. I aim to 'refract' contemporary *uncertainties* about 'the facts of life' through the lens of historic certainties about their biological 'reality' which guided so much anthropological theorising about kinship and conception. By this means, two sets of conception accounts are refracted in and through one another. This two-way traffic, like the work of culture itself, produces new perspectives. The certainties of the past, about a process it is difficult for the most determined constructionist to pick apart – the tenet that it takes a sperm and egg to make a baby – take on a new aspect in light of the 'reality' that for an increasing number of people this equation does not hold. Similarly, the uncertainties about 'assisted conception' in the present, and their contested implications for the future, take on new dimensions in relation to the variety of conception accounts documented and debated by anthropologists in the past, albeit with nothing like the contemporary advent of new reproductive technologies in mind. I argue this refraction is productive, not only as 'a cultural account of assisted conception', but as a theoretical and methodological exercise for late twentieth-century anthropology.

In his trenchant critique of the study of kinship, David Schneider claims that 'kinship has been defined by European social scientists, and European social scientists use their own folk culture as the source of many, if not all, their ways of formulating and understanding the world around them' (1984: 193). This is the definition that produces their 'genealogical amnesia', or what Schneider calls the 'Doctrine of the Genealogical Unity of Mankind', in the form of Eurocentric, *a priori* assumptions about the existence of an object of study (kinship) which may or may not exist everywhere, and which, in any event, cannot usefully be presumed to refer, ultimately, to a genealogical grid. This is the same point Bouquet emphasises *within Europe*, namely that the *ur*-object of 'kinship' is not always 'pedigree'.

The implication is that the pedigree-referent (for that is the meaning of 'genealogy' to which Schneider refers) is *specifically English*, or at least British. Schneider's conclusion is that, unless anthropologists are willing to get rid of kinship altogether, which he advocates, they can only use kinship *as* a European folk model. The anthropologist would thus be armed with the question 'given this [European folk definition of kinship], do these particular people have it or not?' (Schneider, 1984: 200). As a result, he suggests, 'kinship might then become a special custom distinctive of European culture, an interesting oddity at worst, like the Toda bow ceremony' (201).

This study pursues this question somewhat differently. It presumes another option is to apply the distinctive British model of kinship to a distinctively late twentieth-century British kinship dilemma, which is the question of how to make sense of new forms of technological assistance to conception which create new 'relativities' in the space where certain relations once stood. Kinship may indeed be a 'special custom' of European folk culture. But even so, it is very poorly understood, as current uncertainties about its definition clearly indicate. That 'the definition of mother' and 'father' were being debated in the British Parliament at the time of this study is but a superficial indication of the scope of uncertainty and transition occurring in the realm of 'ties established through procreation', which is what kinship has traditionally meant to anthropologists.

The aim of *Embodied Progress* is thus differently comparative from the cross-cultural comparison familiar to anthropology. It aims to open up a scope of ('refractory') comparison *within* the cultural apparatus which makes up anthropology. I argue this dimension of cultural analysis itself comprises an *additional comparative perspective*, which in turn can be put into dialogue with the more traditional forms of anthropological comparison that are ongoing. Hence, this project speaks to the longstanding anthropological aims of elucidating and documenting cultural difference; however, it does so by addressing the question of *what kinds of difference these can be*. It is, I argue, only possible to appreciate the 'scale' of difference imaginable to the anthropologist if we in turn recognise the constitution of that 'scale' itself.

This premise widens the possibilities outlined by Schneider. He emphasised the fixity of the 'genealogical grid' as a point of reference for anthropologists seeking to define 'kinship', and argued that all anthropological definitions of kinship ultimately refer to it in a manner that makes them tautological. Yet, by stressing the givenness of genealogy, Schneider perhaps overstated its 'obviousness'. As Bouquet has shown in her recent work, the pedigree of genealogy *within Europe* is both complex and contradictory (1994, 1995a, 1995b). This point is also emphasised by Strathern, in her discussion of Darwin's use of genealogical analogies in his constitution of 'nature' as a consanguinous unity (1992a).[5] The option, in other words, is not only to presume genealogy as a fixed point of reference, but as an admittedly Eurocentric one (as Schneider suggests). Another option is to acknowledge that even within European, or English, usage, this concept is not as fixed as it appears.

As Bouquet has shown, the history of 'genealogy' in Europe reveals a far more complex picture of this presumed-to-be-self-evident term than has been previously acknowledged. A similar refraction is provided by new technology, which also 'defamiliarises' genealogy. The 'genealogical grid' that is argued to have been such a stable and rigid 'scale' for measuring other cultures' definitions of kinship can be argued itself to be destabilised and denaturalised by new technology. At the root of ideas of coming into being, whether they are defined 'reproductively' or not, has been the idea of vitality. Be it a spirit-child embodying a matrilineal ancestor, or a 'miracle baby' conceived in a test-tube, the notion of 'coming into being' has denoted the creation of new life. This is precisely the aim of much biotechnology: to create new life forms. But in so doing, technological assistance to life itself troubles previous certainties, about descent, relatedness, and kinship. Should children be conceived from the ovaries of aborted fetuses? Should a surrogate mother gestate a fetus that is genetically unrelated to her? Should 'twins' be gestated years apart? It is for these reasons that advances in the sciences of biotechnology engender cultural anxiety about scientists 'playing God' with 'the facts of life'. They are no longer playing by the genealogical grid that was once assumed to be both primordial, 'rimless' and irrevocable.

I argue in the conclusion to this book that kinship theory is an essential tool for understanding such contemporary Euro-American anxieties. Much as 'kinship' may rightly be characterised as an antique European 'folk model', it is none the less valuable for precisely these reasons, as is the rest of 'antique European folk culture'! Though it may seem unfamiliar to be arguing that just-because-its-traditional-doesn't-mean-its-reactionary in the service of proposing what I denominate 'postmodern kinship theory' at the end of this book, this is, in fact, wholly consistent with the most traditional definition of postmodernism itself, namely the redeployment of traditional elements in new configurations.

This is one of several meanings of postmodern kinship theory with which I conclude this book. The new configurations, perspectives and refractions the history of kinship theory can provide are, in my view, multiple, available and necessary. I derive this view as much from my teaching of both graduate and undergraduate anthropology students, in England and in the United States, as I do from my own relationship to anthropology, which, like that of most of my generation, has been composed in equal parts of scepticism and appreciation. Although the 'virgin birth' debates will be familiar ground to readers of an older generation, born in the 1930s and 1940s, they are much less familiar to mine, born in the 1960s and the 1970s. It is for this reason I rehearse this much-travelled ground in what may seem to be redundant detail. This is because I share with other members of my age-cohort who trained in anthropology programs in the 1980s a troubled relationship to its past and future. Although clearly this is not a 'new' phenomenon, it has its own particularities for every generation, and the relationship of current anthropologists to the history of the discipline is an ongoing source of reinventing its future. This too is a reproductive dilemma, and one to which disciplinary technologies are as central a source of confusion as technology has become in other reproductive domains.

Embodied Progress also speaks to a wider audience of readers concerned with the implications of new reproductive and genetic technologies, which have become the source of a burgeoning literature in their own right. I hope it also offers useful insights and analysis for readers with their own experiences of reproductive assistance. In addition, this book contributes to the effort to bridge between anthropology and cultural studies. In particular, it contributes to the cultural analysis of science, which is also an expanding area of scholarship at present. To all of these areas, a concern with gender is central, and though I point to 'kinship' more often than 'gender' *per se* in this account, the centrality to both fields of biological models of reproduction provides a connecting thread I hope will be read as implicit throughout.

I derive my title, *Embodied Progress*, from the specific dilemmas I encountered among women and couples who have undergone assisted conception procedures, and the broader theme of how technological progress, as a cultural value, becomes embodied through reproductive practices. The ongoing development of new life forms through new forms of scientific and technological innovation daily gains momentum: from transgenic and trans-species organisms, to the 'dry' algorithmic 'life' forms of artificial life laboratories, to the imagined recreations of extinct life forms in films such as *Jurassic Park*, to the Human Genome Project which is popularly dubbed 'Man's Second Genesis', to the germline modifications of human hereditary substance now being debated internationally, and the list goes on. With such forms of progress also emerge new uncertainties. Once grounded on the symbolic ground of 'naturalness', which represented 'nature' as a fixed, *a priori* given to which human interventions were always 'after', 'based upon', 'rooted in' or transformative of, human reproduction and the reproductive processes of plants, animals, bacteria and micro-organisms, are increasingly denaturalised by technology. Instead, it is the 'helping hand' of technological assistance, the cultural values of scientific progress and consumer choice, and the imperatives of economic growth which provide the representational ground such reproductive innovations are seen to be 'based upon', 'rooted in', 'after' or determined by. This does not mean reproduction is no longer seen as 'natural': to the contrary, new forms of reproductive technology are ubiquitously re-naturalised. Technology is seen to be 'giving nature a helping hand', as one pamphlet describing the technique of IVF analogises this relationship. None the less, technological progress, consumer choice and economic growth are cultural values which, unlike 'naturalness', convey open-ended malleability and the transcendence of limits. The instrumentalisation of conception described in *Embodied Progress* indexes the changing meanings of 'the facts of life' in such a context. The lived, immediate, and concrete dilemmas produced in one specific set of relations to the enterprising-up of life itself are indicated by the experience of the women and couples interviewed for this book, and it is for what their experiences can reveal about the other myriad variations on this encounter that it is entitled.

Above all, the experiences of women and couples undergoing IVF described here reveal three key components of the encounter with contemporary reproductive medicine. To begin with, a significant discrepancy can be seen to emerge between the representation of IVF as a series of progressive stages and the experience of the procedure (for the majority of couples) as a serial failure to progress. Against the will and determination to progress successfully through the many stages of IVF emerges a continual theme of, often unexplained, failure – such as failure to produce enough eggs, failure of the eggs to fertilise, and so forth. This discrepancy can be seen in terms of a gap between the representation of IVF (as a progress narrative) and the infrequency of success (which occurs on average about 10 per cent of the time).

A second component of the encounter with IVF is the extent to which technological intervention and potential enablement come to define the reproductive process, and to become the focus of intense, preoccupying and often difficult hopes and desires on the part of both IVF clinicians and their clients. The several ways in which repro-duction can be seen to be redefined by the process of becoming technologised, commodified, professionalised and achieved are ex-plored in some depth in this study.

Finally, a consequence of these changes in the reproductive process is the production of new uncertainties. It is one of the central ironies of contemporary reproductive medicine that although the degree of intervention now possible into conception and pregnancy results from increasing confidence, technical sophistication and scientific knowledge, these very interventions increasingly reveal how poorly understood the 'facts of life' remain. For women and couples undergoing IVF, a consequence of the degree of unexplained failure in the context of assisted conception is that the goal of resolution becomes a receding horizon. "We'll just have a go" soon becomes a preoccupying gambit of tantalising prospects ('there is just some minor adjustment to be made') cross-cut by acute dis-appointments and ambiguities ('it could have worked, it should have worked, we really don't know why it didn't work').

It is the complex process whereby the lived, embodied dilemmas of IVF enact a transformative effect upon the women and couples engaged in the pursuit of a 'miracle baby' which is revealed through the vivid narratives of progress and failure related in Chapters 3, 4 and 5. Going into IVF, many women recalled having been motivated by what they initially perceived as a certain resolution to their reproductive uncertainty: either they would succeed, or at least they would have the knowledge that they had exhausted all options. Despite failure being acknowledged as the most likely outcome, even failure was perceived to bring with it a peace of mind that otherwise evaded them.

Unforeseen in such a bid for resolution is the extent to which IVF 'takes over' and becomes 'a way of life'. The unexpected com-plexity, ambiguity and difficulty of the IVF procedure subtly changes the landscape of options into a bewildering array of refinements, adjustments, new procedures and possibilities. The very potential which may have appeared at the outset to be enabling, hopeful and welcome may over time become disabling, stressful and even threatening.

Deciding to abandon hope for success may have become much more difficult after 'living for the dream' from cycle to cycle, often over several years. Against the urge to terminate unsuccessful treatment may be the fear that success is only one step away. Hence, the certainty of resolution – one way or another – which often characterises the decision to undertake IVF can be seen to dissipate over the course of serial failure (which, even for the minority of couples who eventually succeed, most often comprises the better part of their treatment).

Beliefs and hope concerning progress, and the difficulty of 'making sense of misconceptions', thus comprise the antipodes of 'living IVF'. One reason a narrative approach has proven useful to the analysis of conception, and assisted conception, is because of its generic composition out of beginnings and endings, obstacles and resolutions, and the seriality of events. Narrative time recapitulates biological time in its progressive, developmental and cumulative linearity. Temporalised as causal sequences, conception narratives make most sense read backwards, after the fact of successful outcomes. When all of the causal elements are present, but the expected outcome is not realised, an important element of narrativity is lost: it is not clear if the story has ended, there is no resolution, and thus no closure.

Narrative form also structures accounts of scientific progress, which often proceed as stories of discovery, revelation and triumph. Highly gendered, the adventure narratives of scientific progress rely heavily upon the idiom of marching forward into the unknown. The image of scientific pioneers, embarking upon an expedition or voyage of discovery, analogises scientific progress to exploration, conquest and acquisitory penetration into unmapped territory.

Assisted conception thus comprises a densely narrativised cultural practice: from the well-known developmental trajectory of the 'facts of life'; to the post-Darwinian temporalisation of natural history in terms of evolutionary progress; to the progressivist history of modern science; to the depiction of techniques such as IVF in terms of a series of progressive stages.

Ethnographically, that is, from the point of view of the women and couples who encounter IVF as a 'way of life', as participants in the demands of assisted conception procedures, the search for resolutions can be understood as a narrative dilemma: how to reach 'the end of the story' when neither the causality nor seriality of events can be ordered as a progressive sequence?

Like the experiences of so many of the women and couples interviewed for this study, the mode of presentation in this book is not a seamless trajectory, but a series of reframings. Like the broken conception narratives which are its primary objects of study, this account achieves greatest coherence at the post-ultimate moment, that is, upon retrospection. Some patience, therefore, is asked of the reader in negotiating a series of frame-shifts. At the outset, 'Conception among the Anthropologists' considers 'the facts of life' in terms of the classic ethnographic dilemma posed by non-biological conception narratives. Within this frame, 'the facts of life' are considered a scientific certainty among the anthroplogists, and the anthropological dilemma consists of making sense of non-western ('primitive') models of causality and agency through which coming into being is explained. In turn, this very certainty comes to be read as symptomatic of the ethnocentrism towards which late twentieth-century anthropology has become critically self-conscious. Within this frame, then, the 'facts of life' are transformed from a presumed (universal, self-evident, biological and scientific) certainty into an occasion to reveal what that certainty has obscured. In this sense, 'Conception among the Anthropologists' has been refracted through wider debates about science as an authoritative knowledge system, modern biology as a discursive system, and the cultural specificity of anthropology's own representational devices.

The frame shifts rather abruptly in Chapter 2, 'Contested conceptions in the enterprise culture', to Thatcher's Britain in the late 1980s, in which the desire to produce a family acquired very specific cultural meanings as part of a radical redefinition of the nation, the citizen and the body politic. In this context, technological assistance to conception emerges as a distinctive niche market in the increasingly privatised economy of healthcare services. Although reproduction, in plants, animals and micro-organisms as well as humans, has become increasingly technologised, commodified and managed since the 1950s, and although this is in many ways a global or transnational phenomenon, Chapter 2 emphasises the ways in which such transformations always occur as part of specific local, national, and regional cultures. In attempting to identify a specifically British, or English, component to the findings of this study, 'Contested conceptions in the enterprise culture' introduces 'the facts of life' as they are represented, contested and enacted in a specific time and place.

In turn, Chapters 3, 4 and 5 present the results of research based in two British IVF clinics, one public and one private, during the years 1988 and 1989. Organised in relation to the two key themes that emerged out of participant-observation and interviews with twenty-two women and couples, these chapters depict 'the facts of life' in the context of assisted, or achieved (or, more often, not-achieved) conception. Far from a certain, self-evident, scientifically understood or biologically determined causal sequence, conception in the context of IVF emerges as a miraculous, mysterious and unpredictable process. How women and couples come to feel they 'have to try' IVF, how it then 'takes over' and becomes 'a way of life', and how both success and failure become more complicated matters than was initially presumed are some of the important features of achieved conception revealed in these chapters. Very much in contrast with the assumption guiding anthropological accounts of 'Other' cultures' (misconceived) conception models – that is, that it does, in fact, take a sperm and an egg to make a baby, not an ancestral spirit – the world of achieved conception clearly reveals how impoverished is the causal model of conception offered by modern biological science and clinical medicine.

These different frames are brought together in the concluding title chapter with the aim of suggesting numerous connections, contrasts, continuities and disjunctures suggested by the book as a whole. Rather than a denouement, the concluding chapter emphasises the play of certainty and uncertainty surrounding 'the facts of life' in twentieth-century anthropology, and within Euro-American cultural life more broadly. As a distinctive and powerful constellation of beliefs and knowledge concerning origins, development and progress, 'the facts of life' remain a uniquely important site of cultural practice.

As this account is not conventionally anthropological, so it is unconventionally ethnographic. One description of the approach taken here is 'multi-sited ethnography', a practice recently characterised by Marcus as: 'multi-sited research . . . designed around chains, paths, threads, conjunctions, or juxtapositions of locations in which the ethnographer establishes some form of literal, physical presence, with an explicit, posited logic of association or connection among sites that in fact drives the argument of the ethnography' (1995: 105). The drive to establish a logic of connection among sites is paralleled here by the desire to explore a logic of connection among methods, such as those derived from feminist theory, cultural studies, science studies and globalisation theory as well as anthropology. Together, the attempt to respatialise anthropological approaches to culture, and to utilise more interdisciplinary approaches to cultural theory, comprise an effort to contribute to the reworking of contemporary ethnography. Hence, this project did not involve the degree of habitation or dwelling within a community which is often, and rightly, considered the hallmark of a specifically anthropological ethnographic method. However, as Marcus points out, the limitations of a more holistic approach to culture become particularly evident in the context of the more piecemeal, discontinuous, fragmented and incoherent 'lifeworlds' inhabited by participants in, for example, IVF as a 'way of life'. In other words, to use Marcus's formulation, 'multi-sited enthnography ... arises in response to empirical changes in the world and therefore to transformed locations of cultural production. Empirically, following the thread of connection itself impels the move toward multi-sited ethnography' (1995: 97).

As the 'lifeworlds' brought into being among user-groups of reproductive services are constituted across a range of locations, so too is that service sector itself composed of a myriad of intersecting social, professional, financial, governmental and clinical institutions. The effort to provide an 'ethnographic' representation of such a process must also attend to the various local, national and discursive logics or systems in reference to which traditional questions of accommodation and resistance must be understood. Hence, although a degree of ethnographic detail is forfeited in the attempt to offer a qualitatively different method of cultural description – which moves from the history of anthropological theory, to the enterprise culture of Thatcherism, to the media representation of 'desperate' infertile couples, to parliamentary debate of human fertilisation and embryology, to the IVF clinic and into the private sitting rooms of a group of IVF clients – the aim is to reconnect culture, social organisation and individual experience along reconfigured dimensions of scale, perspective and system.

As a contribution to 'multi-sited ethnography', the present exercise must be read as a preliminary innovation. As in most such 'innovative' undertakings, there remain a number of unsatisfactory connections within the overall machinery. Where this account fails to deliver a specificity of ethnographic detail, it is my hope to have compensated with a degree of recombinant possibility roughly equal to the costs of generic deviation. After all, even pedigrees are as much the product of mutation as continuity. In much the same way as my own location in this exercise has often felt awkward, unresolved and unevenly realised, so too are the framings offered in the following chapters notably inconsistent. The framing of the history of anthropological debates about conception is textually-based, composed entirely of formal, academic debate – albeit offered as an exercise in cultural interpretation. In Chapter 2, the frame is, by contrast, widely cast across a range of activities, from the history of the modern life sciences to contemporary public debate of assisted conception in Britain. Chapters 3, 4 and 5, though drawing on sources such as literature from pharmaceutical companies and conversations overheard in the nurses station, primarily consist of descriptions offered by women and couples of their experiences of IVF gained from interviews. Hence, little in the way of the 'thick description' available to a more spatially or communally circumscribed observer is reproduced here, much as such description remains central to the traditional project of anthropology.

Consequently, the form of cultural analysis offered here undertakes to be ethnographic through borrowing, refashioning and innovating rather than through generic imitation or technical conformity. The most important borrowing appears as a sensibility, rather than a technique; for if the methods utilised in this endeavour remain roughly-hewn, the sensibility is conventionally anthropological. Both intellectually and politically, the mode of researching this project is most decidedly ethnographic in its reluctance to adopt a singular, polemical or reductive perspective on the complex business of assisted conception. This is determinedly a project which moves away from the tendency in legal studies, bioethics, feminist criticism and many strands of cultural and science studies to take a position, or to argue for or against particular techniques. My interest lies elsewhere, specifically prior to such judgements, at the level of the effort to make visible the accumulated practices, assumptions and constraints which inform most contemporary assessment and discussion of new reproductive and genetic technologies. It is the different angle of vision, the openness of the ethnographic ear, and the willed naiveté of the ethnographic researcher which provided the enabling disciplinary technology for the account of assisted conceptions provided here.

Chapter 1

Conception among the anthropologists

Our model of the natural differences in the roles of men and women in sexual reproduction lies at the core of our studies of the cultural organization of gender, at the same time that it constitutes the core of the genealogical grid that has defined kinship for us.

(Yanagisako 1985: 1)

INTRODUCTION

One of the central theoretical debates for the study of both gender and kinship concerns the relationship between 'natural' (e.g. physical or biological) and social facts. In gender studies this has taken the form of debates around the significance of 'biological' differences between men and women, particularly in terms of sexuality and reproduction, for the cultural construction of gender. These are the debates, among others, which informed the first feminist anthropological writings of the 1970s which argued that while women's subordination was universal it was not due to 'natural' differences between women and men. Rather it was the set of cultural constructions mapped onto 'the facts of female biology' (Rosaldo and Lamphere 1974b: 8) which, it was argued, was the causal factor behind the 'sexual assymetry [that is] presently a universal fact of social life' (1974b: 3).

This perspective was a significant advance over previous evolutionary and biologically deterministic arguments regarding women's status. In particular, it was an important critique of sociobiological theories which explained female subordination in biologically deterministic terms. The views that women were universally the subordinate sex, and that their subordination was due to their reproductive roles, were (and continue to be) widely used to justify claims that women's subordination is rooted in their biology.

Yet in creating such arguments, feminist anthropologists continued to reinforce a notion of the biological real as a universal given, and as prior to social life. For example, in her famous essay 'Is female to male as nature is to culture', Sherry Ortner argued that '*it is simply a fact* that proportionately more of a woman's body space . . . is taken up with the natural processes surrounding the reproduction of the species' (1974b: 74–5, emphasis added). Although Ortner was able effectively to challenge theories of biological determinism by turning to symbolic and structuralist accounts of culture, her argument relied upon a fixed definition of the 'biological facts' of human reproduction. Like de Beauvoir, on whose claim that the female is 'more enslaved to the species than the male, her animality is more manifest' (cited in Ortner 1974: 74) she modelled her own argument, Ortner did not challenge the seemingly fixed and undeniable significance of the 'biological facts' of reproduction underlying the construction and maintenance of sexual difference.

In the second major anthology of American feminist anthropology to emerge during the 1970s (Reiter 1975), Gayle Rubin proposed a more theoretically sophisticated model for the interrelationship between cultural and 'natural' facts in the structuring of gender and kinship. Rubin's definition of the 'sex/gender system' (1975: 159) through which women are made subordinate 'is the set of arrangements by which a society transforms biological sexuality into products of human activity, and in which these transformed needs are satisfied'. Rubin employed Lévi-Strauss's theory of the exchange of women to describe how the oppression of women is *a product of* kinship arrangements which construct particular 'relationships by which sex and gender are organised and produced' (1975: 177). She then turned to Lacanian psychoanalysis to propose how these kinship systems are reproduced through the 'traces left in the psyches of individuals as a result of their conscription into systems of kinship' (1975: 188). She argued that the theory of the Oedipus Complex is useful to explain how social systems of kinship are structurally mapped onto individual subjectivity, thus serving as an 'apparatus for the production of sexual personality' (1975: 189). This in turn explained the intergenerational transmission of male-dominance and the resulting tenacity of sex and gender roles, much as Nancy Chodorow had done before her (1974). Following Juliet Mitchell, Rubin argued that the 'precise fit' between and Lacanian psychoanalysis and the kinship theory of Lévi-Strauss allows for a profoundly accurate *descriptive* account of both the individual and social reproduction of women's subordination. She was also aware of the danger of this exercise – that 'both psychoanalysis and structuralism are, in one sense, the most sophisticated theories of sexism around' and that 'the sexism of the tradition of which they are a part tends to be dragged in at each borrowing' (1975: 200).

The problem for Ortner, Rubin, Chodorow and others was that the structuralist theories they used to critique biological essentialism themselves relied upon *a priori* constructions of sex and gender difference based upon the 'biological facts' of reproduction. However, the ensuing feminist critique of Ortner and Rubin focused more on the derivative structuralist model of the nature/culture opposition than the prerequisite assumptions about reproduction or sexual difference. Most significantly, the assumption that in all cultures there exists a bipolar opposition between nature and culture was both theoretically and ethnographically challenged as ethnocentric (MacCormack 1980; Goodale 1980; Gillison 1980; Strathern 1980). It was similarly argued that the nature-culture opposition has changed considerably within European culture (Jordanova 1980; Bloch and Bloch 1980) and that it has negotiable meanings elsewhere (Poole 1981; Harris 1980).

In addition to critiquing the nature/culture split, feminist anthropologists argued that women's subordination was not universal. Feminist materialist accounts, roughly following Engels, located women's subordination in the processes of State formation and, in contemporary cultures, the effects of global capitalist penetration (Leacock 1981). According to these arguments, women's traditional power bases in the kinship sector, which had formerly given them equal status to men were, and continue to be, undermined by the colonialist and imperialist practices of male-dominated, western capitalist societies. Thus, the origins of women's subordination are not biological but historical, and the current extent of women's subordination is a modern rather than ancient or prehistoric phenomenon. A related argument proposed that what power women still retain within the kinship sector is invisible from the point of view of western/male-dominated societies, in which women's roles are defined as wives and mothers and devalued (Sacks 1982). Both arguments stressed that women's subordination is not, as Lacanians or structuralists would have it, either original or inevitable in human society.

The critique of biology as a culturally and historically specific belief system supported such arguments. Historians of sexuality and the family such as Foucault (1973, 1976, 1980), Aries (1962), Weeks (1985), Faderman (1981) or Donzelot (1980) documented the importance of the historical emergence of biological definitions of pathology, particularly through medicine and psychiatry, as forms of social control. In particular, the work of Foucault introduced the term 'discourse' through which bodies of knowledge or expertise are linked to regulatory practices of classification and surveillance. The importance of these arguments for gender and kinship studies lies in their identification of biological definitions of pathology as potent sources of cultural formations of personhood, sexuality, the family, and reproduction. In other words, they expose the relationship between science and culture as a changing historical one, with particular implications for our understanding of 'biological facts' and their place in commonsense western definitions of sexuality, procreation, gender and kinship[1]. From an anthropological perspective, they provided substantiation for the claims of those, such as Schneider (1984), who argued that the models of kinship produced by European anthropologists reproduced a European ethno-epistemology derivative of folk concepts such as genealogy, pedigree or descent lines.

This re-evaluation of the very terms which structured the initial debates in feminist anthropology about the relationship between 'natural facts' and the cultural construction of gender opened up a whole new set of questions (see Butler 1990 and Haraway 1991 for excellent reviews of these debates). No longer could a universal dichotomy of nature/culture be assumed. Nor was it possible to argue that women's subordination was either an original or a universal fact of human social life. Neither was it any longer meaningful simply to refer to 'the facts of female biology' because it was no longer evident what, if any, explanatory significance these 'facts' alone have to offer. The challenge became one of moving beyond the basic categories which structured the debates about gender, kinship, sexuality and reproduction – in particular the dichotomous constructions of male/female, nature/culture, culture/biology, natural facts/social facts that limited the scope of inquiry in the past.

Yet, while this recognition of the need to escape the clutches of host of obfuscating binarisms has been argued since the early 1980s, and although a wealth of alternatives now exist to such formulations, the legacy of the distinction between 'natural facts' and social facts remains a powerful epistemic tradition which is not easily displaced. It continues to be the case that the 'biological facts of human reproduction', or 'the facts of life' occupy a privileged explanatory status in relation to many core questions of social organisation and cultural change. Particularly in the context of a resurgence of biological, and especially genetic, essentialism in the 1990s, it can appear that a certain amount of headway has been lost, or lost track of. This difficulty reflects the seemingly intransigent depth of purchase the idea of culture and society being 'after', or 'based on', or 'rooted in' the facts of nature, genetics or biology continues to exercise in Euro-American social theory (Schneider 1984; Strathern 1992a). My contribution here attempts to offer further elaboration on this important theme with the aid of the 'defamiliarising' lens provided by new reproductive and genetic technology.[2]

In this chapter, my focus is broadly aimed at the conceptual history informing the theorisation of kinship, gender and reproduction in modern American and British social anthropology. However, my chosen exemplification of these broad areas is the analysis of conception theories. I mean by this specifically the debates in anthropology surrounding 'folk models' of reproduction, or more specifically 'the facts of life'. I argue in this chapter that the rich and illuminating history of twentieth-century anthropological debates about conception theory, in particular the so-called 'virgin birth' debates, yields specific historical evidence about the potent operations of the idea of 'biological facts' within anthropological theory. In turn, the focus can be widened back out again to trace the implications from one specific area of theoretical debate (conception theories) to broader questions of social organisation, such as kinship, gender and reproduction.

'IN THE BEGINNING. . . .':
ANTHROPOLOGY AND THE 'FACTS OF LIFE'

From its inception, the anthropological investigation of kinship has been centred around the social organisation and regulation of so-called biological facts such as procreation and genetic relatedness or 'consanguinity'. It was the discovery of classificatory kinship terms which did not correspond to 'true' genetic relationships which led early kinship theorists in the nineteenth century to hypothesise a system of group marriage and 'primitive promiscuity' out of which more 'advanced' kinship systems had evolved. 'Classificatory' systems referred to the social definition of kinship, as distinct from 'descriptive' systems which corresponded to the 'real' or 'accurate' rendering of biological-relatedness, or, what Lewis Henry Morgan (1871) described as both the 'natural system', or the 'system of consanguinity'. Significantly, therefore, these models applied to social organisation the analogy so central to Darwin's model, of nature as a consanguinous system. This perspective on kinship was shared by many early-twentieth century anthropologists, including Rivers (1910, 1924), Frazer (1910), and Hartland (1909). It was a perception that derived from the European scientific assumption that kinship categories should be read directly from 'blood' ties as a matter of commonsense, and that to do otherwise could only be interpreted as ignorance of paternity, or general lack of intellectual development.

Malinowski was among the first anthropologists to provide substantial ethnographic ('scientific') evidence that both sexuality and parenthood were highly structured among 'primitive' peoples, and that they were not merely mistaken, confused, immoral, or less intelligent than Europeans. In his writings on both Australian aborigines and Trobriand Islanders, Malinowski established distinctions between sexuality and procreation, and between procreation and parenthood. The force of Malinowski's argument lay in the fact that both Australian aborigines and Trobriand Islanders claimed to be ignorant of physiological paternity. This discovery greatly weakened the argument that 'promiscuity' prevented the establishment of fatherhood and therefore of individual families (an evolutionary assumption that more properly belonged to the late-nineteenth century, but which persisted well into the early twentieth). In contrast to this view, Malinowski demonstrated that biology was not the basis for paternity among the Trobrianders, thus exposing the ethnocentrism of previous assumptions that paternity could only be defined biologically. By establishing a distinction between social fatherhood and biological fatherhood (originally formulated by Van Gennep 1906, after Durkheim), Malinowski introduced a model of 'natural and social facts' through which to understand kinship systems.

In turn, British social anthropology came to rely on this dual model of kinship, as composed of social and natural elements. Functionalism emphasised the importance of kinship in the realisation of certain fundamental ('psycho-biological') human needs for survival, continuing to demonstrate a preoccupation with marriage, family and sexual arrangements as had the evolutionary theorists whose models they dispatched. Within structural-functionalism, kinship came to be seen as the most important institution for so-called 'simple' societies, and the importance of descent groups, or lineages, was linked to the organisation of kinship, or family, in the theorisation of society as composed of domestic and jural domains.

Since Malinowski, anthropological analyses of kinship have continued to wrestle with the relationship between natural and social facts. Some kinship theorists have continued to use an explicitly biological model to explain kinship, gender, sexuality and reproduction (e.g. Barnes 1961, 1964, 1973; Fortes 1969; Fox 1967). These theorists tended towards a sociobiological or evolutionary perspective, situating the mother–child bond as the 'obvious' proto-social unit, and interpreting kinship in terms of 'reproductive strategies'. Other anthropologists have argued it is meaningless to interpret kinship in terms of biological determinism because biology has no meaning outside of its cultural context (Scheffler and Lounsbury 1971; Schneider 1984). The interrelationship between biological reproduction and social reproduction within specific cultural and historical contexts is the focus of these arguments.

Schneider was an important figure in these debates because he has both analysed the history of kinship theory in terms of its privileging of 'biological' facts (1984), and provided ethnographic insights on the role of biology as a symbolic system (1968b). Schneider claimed that all kinship theorists have implicitly assumed a biological model as their guide, even when they have claimed otherwise. 'The Doctrine of Genealogical Unity of Mankind' is Schneider's gloss on the seemingly intractable tendency to assume the 'biological facts' of reproduction as the basis for kinship theory (1984: 119). These and other components of his arguments about the role of 'biology' in anthropological explanation are described in more detal in a later section of this chapter devoted to his work.

Schneider's claims coincided with the concerns of many feminist anthropologists, for whom the 'biological facts of human reproduction' were also a central point of contention. In her powerful critique of Schneider, Yanagisako identified this essential link, arguing that Schneider overlooked important implications of his own argument. As she stated in her 1985 paper, 'The Elementary Structure of Reproduction in Kinship and Gender Studies':[3]

My argument is that the model of sexual procreation, which Schneider contends defines the field of kinship studies, also defines the field of gender studies; consequently, what we have treated as two distinct, if intimately connected, domains of study in anthropology, are more accurately viewed as two aspects of a single domain defined by the same cultural model. Our model of the natural difference in the roles of men and women in sexual reproduction lies at the core of our studies of the cultural organization of gender, at the same time that it constitutes the core of the genealogical grid that has defined kinship for us.

(Yanagisako 1985: 1)

Rather than being taken-for-granted as the basis for both kinship and gender, Yanagisako argues it is the 'biological facts' of reproduction and sexual difference which *most need to be explained*. As she and Jane Collier later expressed this view, 'we argue that gender and kinship have been defined as fields of study by our folk conception of the same thing, namely, the biological facts of reproduction' (Collier and Yanagisako 1987b: 15).

An important implication of this argument is that the 'folk model' of the 'biological facts of reproduction' is itself a cultural product of Euro-American social theory, and, in that sense, artefactual. It is for this reason that the 'folk conception' of conception itself comprises an important chapter in the history of Euro-American social theory. The timeliness of revisiting the significance of anthropological debates about the conception theories of other cultures is underscored by the renewed uncertainty about the 'facts of life' within contemporary Euro-American societies as a result of new reproductive technologies, which have, like the anthropological project itself, 'made the familiar strange'. It is my overriding aim in this book to put these various 'conceptions' in dialogue with one another. By offering both a history of anthropological debates about conception, and a culturally grounded account of their contemporary renegotiation, a specific two-way traffic is explored: past chapters in anthropological debate yield new insights into contemporary uncertainties, and new technology provides a different lens through which to view the certainties of past debates.

THE VIRGIN BIRTH DEBATES

The remainder of this chapter reviews the debates concerning what came to be known as 'virgin birth', referring to the so called 'ignorance of physiological paternity' which has been central to the evolution of anthropological theory. This is thus an exercise which extends Yanagisako's argument by situating contemporary debates about 'the facts of life' in relation to the 'folk European' categories out of which they emerged. Particularly the role of biological science as itself a 'folk European' preoccupation is clearly revealed in the extent to which it has so pervasively influenced anthropological theories and methods. The history outlined here references the broader question of the significance of 'biology' as a concept in anthropology and the human sciences.

My focus highlights how subsequent generations of anthropologists have theorised the relationship between 'the biological facts of human reproduction' and culture in relation to the debates about 'virgin birth'. Giving undeservedly short shrift to the very long history of anthropological debates about paternity in this introductory section (below), I begin more detailed discussion in the early-twentieth century with Malinowski's work on the Trobrianders and the debates his ethnographic findings generated among anthropologists. In the subsequent sections I discuss the arguments of Edmund Leach, Melford Spiro, David Schneider and Annette Weiner with particular attention to how their accounts of conception and procreation affect their models of kinship. I return to the argument proposed by Yanagisako, and the work of other feminist anthropologists on reproduction in the conclusion, which reviews the state of current debate about the significance of 'biological facts' an anthropology.

As both Delaney (1986, 1991) and Coward (1983) illustrate, debates about conception have a privileged place in the history of anthropology. From the late-nineteenth century onwards, 'accurate' knowledge of physical paternity served as a primary measure of progress towards civilisation. According to the evolutionary view, the difference between barbarity and civility was precisely indexed by knowledge of 'the facts of life'. As noted above, 'correct' knowledge of physical paternity was read as evidence of the triumph of intellect and reason over the hindrances of instinct, animality and savagery. Knowledge of paternity, or its stated absence, was a preoccupation of early anthropologists for whom it functioned as a signifier of intellectual, social, moral and political development.

Writing in the mid-1800s, Bachofen proposed a direct challenge to the arguments of Henry Maine concerning the role of the patriarchal family (1861). In contrast to Maine's account of the complex

governmental role of the patriarchal family in early society, Bachofen proposed an evolutionary model that was to become widely
influential. Society, he argued, arose not out of the *patria potestas*
presumed by Maine, or his predecessors such as Robert Filmer
(1630), but out of a series of significant transitions in sexual,
reproductive and conjugal arrangements. The history of society,
Bachofen argued, was not the history of the patriarchal (Biblical)
family as it expanded to become a wider set of organising structures.
Instead, this history was one of radical transitions separating one era
from the next, much as the waves of extinction evident from natural
history indexed sweeping changes over time.

According to Bachofen, society arose out of maternal instinct. The
nurture towards children derivative of the biological requirements of
maternity produced the basis for the first societies, which were
matriarchal, and characterised by what he called 'mother-right'.
Mater semper certa est, the saying went: motherhood is always
certain, and by reason of its obviousness, it was presumed to exercise
a greater role in primitive society. In the matriarchal societies
envisaged by Bachofen, the principles were the exact opposite of
those arising with the triumph of 'father-right' in an epochal battle
of the sexes, postulated as the origin of the modern social order.
Under mother- right, the left hand had prominence over the right, the
moon over the sun, the emotion over the intellect, and sentiment over
reason. All of these features were seen to derive from women's
reproductive role in bearing and raising children, which caused her
to be religiously-minded, sensuous and irrational.

The triumph of father-right and of the modern, civilised character
of society resulted from the historic overthrow of the ancient
matriarchate by the patriarchal order. Relying upon classical literature, ancient mythology, and traveller's accounts of so-called
'primitive' societies, Bachofen chronicled the transformation by
which the matriarchal order was defeated, thereafter to be sub-
ordinated and repressed. Critical to this transition was the discovery
of physical paternity. Whereas the relation of mother to child was
seen to be self-evident, the relation of a father to his offspring was
considered abstract, intangible and non-obvious. Whereas the mother
could know her offspring by the sensuous, bodily perception of a
physical tie, the discovery of the paternal tie required intellect and
deductive reason. Hence, the triumph of father-right, founded on the
triumph of intellect over sensuousness, instantiated the modern
privileging of mind over body, reason over nature, and man over

woman. In these accounts, paternity was assumed to be possessive, and knowledge of paternity a rational achievement driven by the need to deduce the basis of this possessive relationship. It is above all the enormous scope of what was presumed to be consequent upon the deductive mastery of the 'facts of life' in relation to the 'physical' ties of fatherhood which these early debates make evident.

Though by contemporary standards fanciful and unscholarly, the influence of Bachofen's evolutionary model was profound, and symptomatic of the broad shift towards developmental accounts of human and natural history in the mid-nineteenth century, out of which Darwinism eventually emerged. Following Bachofen, Morgan placed considerable importance upon the unfolding of distinct stages in human social evolution, beginning with the ancient matriarchate, or the matrilineal *gens*. During this stage, a state of 'primitive promiscuity' rendered paternity indecipherable. Morgan hypothesised that primitive groups able to impose some sort of marriage restriction, or prohibition on reproductive selection, gained greater survival advantages. Increasing prohibitions led to the emergence of marriage and monogamy, according to Morgan, who relied heavily on North American Indian societies for his materials. In conjunction with the accumulation of private property, paternity was established as a means of ensuring the heriditary transmission of wealth.

Although Morgan had no specific model of paternity, assuming only that it was in men's self-interest eventually to discover the physical basis of their relation to children, this discovery was essential to his argument. It was equally important to Engels, who, dedicating his book to Morgan, consolidated the evolutionary view of social progress in his classic text *On the Origin of the Family, Marriage, Private- Property and the State*. Deftly remobilising Morgan's argument to do service for an account of the emergence of capitalism, Engels squarely located its origin in sexual politics. In neatly outlined stages, Engels chronicled the transition of society from primitive promiscuity, through matrilineal society, culminating in the 'world historic defeat of the female sex' occasioned by the discovery of physical paternity (1884).

The question of physical paternity remained a prominent theme, even an obsession, in early anthropological writings during the late-nineteenth and early-twentieth centuries. Frazer was preoccupied with the question of paternity, and considered totemism to be the result of primitive ignorance of 'the facts of life' (1910). In *The History of Human Marriage* (1891), Westermarck put forward a model of the procreative unit as the basis for the family and society, instigating a challenge to the presumption of procreative ignorance. This followed in part from McLennan's arguments, in which he coined the term 'exogamy' and postulated that knowledge of paternity arose from the custom of fathers giving gifts to children (1865). As debate continued to surround the significance of the family to the emergence of civilised society, an increasing amount of evidence from cultures around the world was available on which to base more detailed speculation.

The publication in 1899 of Spencer and Gillen's *The Native Tribes of Central Australia*, containing a detailed account of aboriginal people's professed ignorance of the relationship between coitus and pregnancy, provided the occasion for renewed interest in the physical paternity question. For commentators such as Westermarck, for whom the procreative function of the family was its primary defining feature, such evidence was difficult to accept. 'I must confess that I have some doubts as to the present existence of any savage tribe where childbirth is considered to be completely independent of sexual intercourse', he wrote (1922: 293). Malinowski, his student, agreed: the expression of ignorance, or as it was then called 'nescience', of physiological paternity corresponded to an imperfect knowledge which was deliberately maintained to preserve the dominant cultural ethos of a group. Nonetheless, for Malinowski 'the question of primitive nescience of paternity' was no less than 'the most exciting and controversial issue in the comparative science of man' (1937: xxiii). It was a question which not only invoked broad questions of kinship social organisation, but of psychology, mythology, religion, technology and knowledge. In addition, this question stood at the heart of controversies about the nature of anthropological investigation, ethnographic interpretation and cross-cultural comparison.

Writing in 1937, Ashley Montagu compiled a compendious study of the procreative beliefs of native Australian peoples, long considered to be among the most 'primitive' of tribal groups, entitled *Coming Into Being Among the Australian Aborigines*. Undertaken at the behest of Westermarck and Malinowski, this study aimed to put to rest the question of professed ignorance of paternity. He concluded 'that in Australia practically universally, according to orthodox belief, pregnancy is regarded as causally unconnected with intercourse' (1937: 207). This was declared by Malinowski, in his introduction to the volume, to be 'the ultimate conclusion of science

. . . supported by an irrefutable body of solid fact' (1937: xxiv). But this was not the end of the story. Debate continued to surround the question of how societies that demonstrated sophisticated knowledge of their environments, could navigate the seas, and possessed detailed zoological knowledge, could remain 'ignorant' of something as 'obvious' as physical paternity?

In the late 1960s, debate flared again in response to Edmund Leach's acerbic 'Virgin Birth' lecture, delivered to the Royal Anthropological Institute in London, in which he took issue with the work of Melford Spiro, and denounced any anthropologists who believed that Australian aboriginals or Trobriand Islanders were truly ignorant as racists (1967). Spiro replied in a lengthy article in *Man*, agreeing with Leach that neither the Trobrianders nor the Australian aborigines could possibly be ignorant, but offering a different, psychoanalytic, account of their claims of being so (1968). The pages of *Man* carried extensive correspondence from other commentators, and so the paternity question again emerged at the heart of debates about such core features of the anthropological project as the interpretation of ethnographic data, the use of cross-cultural comparison, and the analytic frameworks employed to theorise culture and society.

CONCEPTIONS OF CONCEPTION RECONCEIVED

Reviewing the history of anthropological debate concerning theories of conception, it becomes clear that they have held a profound and specific importance in relation to questions about knowledge, as well as sexuality and reproduction. On the one hand, the 'virgin birth' debates are about the discovery of peoples who claimed to be 'ignorant of physiological paternity' (Roth 1903; Spencer and Gillen 1899). The ethnographic facts related to this discovery are themselves the object of debate for one strand in the multiple and interwoven controversies about this issue. Other strands of this debate are about more abstract theoretical questions, such as the meaning of cultural beliefs, the interpretation of ethnographic facts, the relationship between physical and social facts, the relationship between kinship and procreation, and the meaning of 'biological facts' in cross-cultural perspective.

As a result of the many and various agendas attached to the 'virgin birth' debates, there are often differences of opinion about whether the specific issue is 'ignorance of physiological paternity', to use the original historical formulation (Roth 1903), 'parthenogenesis' (Spiro 1968: 249), 'the fertilizing virtue of seminal fluid' and thus 'the real generative power of the sexual act' (Malinowski 1927b: 49); or 'the precise details of the physiology of sex' (Leach 1967: 40). There are differences of opinion as well at the other end of the spectrum, about what the 'virgin birth' debates concern anthropologically. In the words of Malinowski, 'we are really opening up a number of definitely empirical questions referring to the cultural transformation of the biological elements, sex, maternity and fatherhood' (1962: 59). According to Leach, the problem is primarily a methodological one: 'What is really at issue is the technique of anthropological comparison which depends in turn upon the kind of "meaning" which we are prepared to attribute to ethnographic evidence' (1967: 40). Spiro agreed: '[This] controversy is theoretical and methodological in character. It involves such issues as the nature of culture, how it works, what its functions are, what explanatory variables must be attended to in attempting to interpret any of its manifestations' (1968: 243).

As the wide spectrum of these views as to what the 'virgin birth' debates were 'about' makes clear, conceptions of conception among both anthropologists and the peoples they have studied comprise an exemplary chapter in the history of anthropological theory.[4] In turn, by reviewing the arguments of a selected number of participants in this ongoing controversy, it is possible to appreciate the breadth of anthropological concern with the 'biological facts of human reproduction' both over time, and in the present. For each of the theorists discussed below, the 'biological facts' presumed to be so self-evident as to exercise a singular driving force in the history of society come to represent quite distinct forms of knowledge, with specific implications for the study of culture as a whole.

Malinowski: pure biology vs. total culture

It seems hardly necessary to emphasise that for physiological consanguinity *as such* pure and simple, there is no room in sociological science.

(Malinowski 1913: 177)

Malinowski rejected the assumption that the natural and therefore original form of the human family was patriarchal – an orthodox Judaeo-Christian belief supported by both Henry Maine (1861) and

Fustel de Coulanges (1871). In his first published monograph, *The Family Among Australian Aborigines*, Malinowski argued that the family was more 'deeply rooted in social conditions' (1913: 293) than in biology; and, if anything, based on the 'physiological facts' of maternity rather than paternity:

> It is clear that the position of the father is . . . first established socially only, as the husband of the children's mother. . . . The existence of the individual family as a social unit [is] based upon the physiological facts of maternity, the social factor of marriage and other social factors.
>
> (1913: 173)

Malinowski also rejected the arguments of Bachofen (1861), Morgan (1871), McLennan (1886), Frazer (1910) and others who postulated the existence of a matriarchal stage in human history involving group marriage and primitive promiscuity which eventually gave way to the patriarchal nuclear family. Wary of abstract, universalistic analytical models ('armchair anthropologists'), and equally suspicious of theories unsupported by sufficient empirical data, Malinowski energetically challenged the validity of the diffusionist or, so called, 'historical' school with its 'superficial emphasis on material facts' (Leach 1957: 121). Against these theories, Malinowski advocated a method of determined and meticulous empiricism for which he believed there was no substitute, and which was in turn destined to become his own personal hallmark in the production of a fully 'scientific' anthropology (see Firth 1957; Fortes 1957; Weiner 1976).

In addition to these general aspects of Malinowski's background informing his discussions of 'virgin birth' was the significance of his attitude towards 'primitive' peoples. Though it has been rightly argued his views were both contradictory and inconsistent on this account (Leach 1957), Malinowski did openly criticise the 'European point of view' of anthropologists who assumed culturally specific (Victorian) family forms to be superior, thereby justifying their use as interpretive frames of reference (Malinowski 1962: 56). He argued firstly on an epistemological level against the monolithic models of causality and determinism in these theories and claimed that the very questions to which they were addressed were 'irrelevant and fictitious' (1962: 56). Secondly, he objected, on what might be described as more humanitarian grounds, to the missionary view of 'primitive' peoples as 'lawless, inhuman and savage' (1922: 10). To the contrary, argued Malinowski:

Modern science shows ... that their social institutions have a very definite organisation, that they are governed by authority, law and order in their public and personal relations, while the latter are, besides, under the control of extremely complex ties of kinship and clanship.

(1922: 10)

This emphasis on 'scientific' methodology as an antidote to the inaccuracies and racism of prevailing theories, along with his sensitivity to the overemphasis on biological paternity by anthropologists from patriarchal cultures (1962: 56), provide something of an historical context in which to situate Malinowski's distinctive contribution to the study of kinship.

All of these factors were made manifest in Malinowski's thesis, published as *The Family Among Australian Aborigines*, and clearly the product of his training in England under Westermarck and Hobhouse (1913). Many of what were later to be recognised as his most significant contributions to the study of kinship originally appeared in this first monograph. The emphasis on the distinction (first formulated by Van Gennep 1906) between physical parenthood and social parenthood; the recognition of the significance of beliefs about conception in the delineation of kinship systems; the understanding of kinship systems as inextricable from their total cultural context; an attention to the quotidian features of kinship activity we now call social reproduction; and a recognition of the discrepencies between recognised social codes and actual individual behaviour are some of the definitive Malinowskian insights present in this early, text-based research manuscript.

Over and above these factors, the most significant theoretical argument from this volume concerns the meaning and significance of biological facts. Malinowski was unhesitating in his assessment and unwavering in his conclusion that *biological facts do not determine social facts*. Biological relatedness does not determine social relatedness; biological parenthood does not determine social parenthood; physiological paternity does not determine social fatherhood – in short, natural facts do not determine social facts according to Malinowski (1913: 177–9). There is no place in sociological theory for purely physiological facts, he argued, they have no meaning in and of themselves. 'It seems hardly necessary to emphasise that for physiological consanguinity *as such*, pure and simple, there is no room in sociological science' (1913: 177 fn.).

Rather, he insisted, kinship must be understood as a combination of physiological, psychological and sociological processes, and as such must be seen and understood in relation to the total cultural context (1913: 182).[5]

In explicit opposition to the views of earlier anthropologists concerning the axiomatic importance of biological paternity, Malinowski insisted that there is no such thing as a 'physiological fact' *per se* in human social life, or for that matter, outside natural science at all. He insisted that the facts of physiology have no deterministic influence, on either kinship or parenthood, and that instead they are shaped by their cultural context. This was substantiated by his argument that even something as 'obvious', 'natural', and 'biological' as parenthood can be constructed quite differently in different cultures (1913: 180). In part, this insistence derives its force from Malinowski's disdain for the elaborate speculations of his predecessors, for whom a single 'natural fact', such as paternity, could be attributed such disproportionate influence. It is also a sign of his attempt to improve upon Westermarck's theories, in which the procreative function of the nuclear family operated as a kind of unexplained telos.

Somewhat contradictorily, and in spite of his rejection of paternity as an all-important 'biological fact', his views on maternity were clearly biologically-based. He argued until the end of his career, for example, that 'the foundations of the human family are to be found in *the biological fact* of maternity' (1937: xxvi, emphasis added). Hence, although it is necessary to acknowledge the critique of natural facts espoused by Malinowski, it is important not to overstate the case. As a functionalist, he believed certain fundamental 'psychobiological' needs were met by the social order, and the post-Darwinian reproductive telos that informed the work of earlier social theorists of whom he was explicitly critical remained central to the Malinowskian models of culture and society.[6]

Malinowski's account of the Trobriander's theory of conception and gestation begins with their beliefs about death and reincarnation. When a person dies, her or his spirit goes to the island of Tuma to live with other ancestral spirits or *Baloma* (1922: 170; see also 1916). It is from Tuma that all new human life is derived, through a process of reincarnation:

[W]hen a spirit becomes tired of constant rejuvenation, when he has led a long existence 'underneath,' as the natives call it, he may want to return to earth again; and then he leaps back in age and becomes a small preborn infant.

(1922: 171)

Malinowski's informants differed on the exact means whereby the spirit-child (usually called *waywaya*, 'small child' or *pwapwawa*, meaning 'newborn', or simply *gwadi*, meaning 'child' (1922: 177)) reaches the woman's womb. Most accounts agreed that the spirit-child entered the woman's body as 'blood on the head' (1922: 188), 'with which is associated the idea of an effusion of blood, first to the head and then into the abdomen' (1922: 174).

> The spirit-child is laid by the bringer on the woman's head. Blood from her belly rushes there, and on this tide of blood the baby gradually descends until it settles in the womb. The blood helps to build the body of the child – it nourishes it. That is the reason why, when a woman becomes pregnant, her menstrous flow stops.
>
> (1922: 175)

Informants also gave conflicting versions of how the spirit-children appeared and what material form they took, some believing they looked like tiny fetuses or 'like mice', while others claimed they were like tiny children, 'and that they are sometimes very beautiful' (1922: 177).

The ethnographies provided by Malinowski and those of other observers confirm a general association between *sea water* and *conception* among the Trobrianders. Malinowski's informants reported that both the rejuvenation process of ancestral spirits (*Baloma*) on Tuma and their reincarnation as spirit-children involve sea water:

> In the first account of rejuvenation which I obtained in Omarakana, I was told that the spirit 'goes to the beach and bathes in salt water'. . . . Likewise in the final rejuvenation, which makes them return to the infant state, the spirits have to bathe in salt water, and, when they become babies again, they go into the sea and drift. They are always spoken of as floating on drift logs, or on the leaves, boughs, dead sea weed, sea-scum and other light substances which litter the surface of the sea.
>
> (1929: 172–3)

Malinowski also learned that among coastal peoples young girls will not enter sea water that is too cluttered by debris for fear they will conceive (1929: 175). He also reports that 'in villages on the northern coast, there is a custom of filling a wooden baler with water from the sea which is then left overnight in the hut of a woman who wishes to conceive, on the chance that a spirit-child might have been caught in the baler and transfer itself during the night into the woman' (1929: 175–6). On the basis of these and other observations it has been further argued that a woman's water bottles represent her fertility and her sexuality (Wilson 1969: 286–8).[7]

However, these logistical details were not as important to Malinowski as the three main facts of Trobriander beliefs about conception: that 'these rejuvenated spirits, these little pre-incarnated babies or spirit-children, are *the only source from which humanity draws its new supplies of life*' (1929: 171, emphasis added); that 'a pre-born infant finds its way back to the Trobriands and into the womb of some woman, *but always of a woman who belongs to the same clan and sub-clan as the spirit-child itself*' (1929: 171, emphasis added); and that 'the only reason and the real cause of every birth is spirit activity' (1929: 172). The intervention of a controlling spirit is the key element in conception. Though a woman may dream of becoming pregnant and then learn that she is so, it is the agency of the controlling spirit which has caused her to conceive. 'A *baloma* is the real cause of childbirth!' (1929: 174), insisted Malinowski's informants.[8]

Malinowski noted that the Trobianders possessed detailed knowledge of the anatomy of humans and animals, and that they had 'an extensive vocabulary for the various parts of the human body and for the internal organs' (1929: 164). 'The custom of *post mortem* dissections of corpses, and visits among their overseas cannibal neighbours supply them with an exact knowledge of the homologies of the human and animal organisms' (1929: 165), he argued. However, he also claimed that 'their physiological views are crude', 'remarkably defective' and that 'there are many notable gaps in their knowledge about the functions of the most important organs' (1929: 165). Specifically, he found that the Trobrianders have no word for the ovaries, and do not recognise the physiological function of the testes (1929: 168). Both the testes and menstrual blood are regarded as apparel, as decoration or ornamentation, rather than as functional in the physiological sense (1927b: 25–7, 1929: 168–9).

Malinowski's theory of kinship is well demonstrated by his interpretation of the Trobrianders' procreation beliefs – or, as it came to be called, their belief in 'virgin birth'. Kinship was closely connected to procreation in Malinowski's view – indeed so much so that he even suggested kinship should be renamed 'The Procreative Institution' (1962: 57) because of how much he believed a culture's beliefs about the male and female contributions to procreation revealed about their kinship ethos. He argued that 'the respective contributions of the male and of the female parent to the body of the offspring, as estimated in the traditional lore of a given society, form the nucleus of the system of reckoning kinship' (1927b: 7). He argued that both kinship and procreation were concerned with the same set of facts – 'the facts of life' – which he described as 'a number of definitely empirical questions referring to the cultural transformation of the biological elements, sex, maternity and fatherhood' (1962: 59).[9]

Although Malinowski did much to overturn previous assumptions about the relationship of biology to culture, he still worked within that dichotomous framework in theorising his ethnographic data. This caused a certain amount of confusion. Even in his later works Malinowski argues on the one hand for a biological model of maternity (it is the 'more obvious fact in the propagation of species' 1962: 60) and a cultural one ('maternity is thus determined in anticipation by a whole cultural apparatus of rules and prescriptions' (1962: 61)). The evolutionism of his views is also apparent in his accounts of Trobriand 'folk biology'. His extensive attention to beliefs about the body and bodily substances might well have provided an alternative framework through which to view 'biology'. Instead, like previous anthropologists who viewed a lack of knowledge of physical paternity as evidence of 'backwardness', Malinowski compared the Trobriander's 'crude' ideas about the body to western scientific theories, albeit emphasising that they had got the gist of it correctly.

In relation to the question of ignorance of physiological paternity, Malinowski insisted upon two primary points of explanation. He argued first of all that assertions of the non-existence of either physical paternity or maternity upheld the central principle of Trobriand social organisation, namely the continuity of the matrilineal clan structure. Secondly, he argued that although the Trobrianders denied physical paternity *per se*, they were aware of the basic facts concerning the relationship between coitus and pregnancy. 'The so-called primitive ignorance of physiological paternity', he wrote, 'is nothing else but a very imperfect knowledge that intercourse is a necessary though not sufficient condition of the woman being "opened up" as my Trobriand friends put it' (1937: xxxi). Hence, while affirming the ethnographic fact of stated ignorance of either physiological maternity or paternity, Malinowski none the less reconstructed the statements of his informants to render their understandings commensurate with the 'actual facts', albeit 'crudely'.

Contemporary anthropological work on conception beliefs in New Guinea (Jorgensen 1983; Weiner 1976, 1978, 1979) has elaborated upon many of Malinowski's findings, and it is a testament to the thoroughness of his ethnographic observations that they have continued to provide such a rich empirical base for later researchers. This work has also demonstrated the lasting significance of Malinowski's insights into the centrality of conception and procreation beliefs, and beliefs about the body, for understanding the cultural construction of kinship and gender. Indeed, the importance of these insights could not be better demonstrated by the current debates over the definition of procreation and conception currently being waged in response to new reproductive technologies. In these debates, Malinowski's claim that what a society believes about conception can reveal what they believe about everything else is well demonstrated, as is his prescient suggestion that: 'It would be interesting if the sociologist would turn to [our own] societies and make as minute a study of their over-emphasis on paternity as . . . others have made of its disregard in Australia. I venture to foretell that . . . knowledge in the scientific sense is as much affected by cultural elements and reinterpretations as is the case in Australia' (1937: xxxii).

Leach: the question of ignorance and scientific truth

If we put the so-called primitive beliefs alongside the sophisticated ones and treat the whole lot with equal philosophical respect we shall see that they constitute a set of variations around a common structural theme, the metaphysical topography of the relationship between gods and men.

(Leach 1967: 34)

In his Henry Myers lecture of 1967 entitled 'Virgin Birth', Edmund Leach expressed three main concerns in relation to the historic controversy over 'the facts of life'. He argued that:

1 neither the Trobrianders nor the Australian aborigines were ignorant of the facts of physiological paternity;
2 the fact that anthropologists ever believed they were only revealed
   their 'prejudice about ignorance and primitiveness' (1967: 39);
   and,
3 the real problems raised by this controversy have to do with
   method and *belief.*

Leach's argument reformulated the issue of 'biological and social
facts' as one of ignorance vs knowledge, in turn setting up a different
but related dichotomy of cultural dogma vs scientific truth. The
premise of this formulation was Leach's own dogmatic assertion that
it was 'highly improbable *on common sense grounds* that genuine
"ignorance" of the basic facts of physiological paternity should
anywhere be a cultural fact' (1967: 41, emphasis added). In defence
of this assertion, he argued that there are only a very few groups who
allegedly do not know the 'facts of physiological paternity'; that
these exceptional groups are not isolated from other peoples who 'do
know' but are often in close contact with them; and that 'human
beings . . . have displayed a collective problem solving intelligence
of an astoundingly high order' and, everywhere 'display an almost
obsessional interest in matters of sex and kinship' (1967: 41).
Therefore, he concluded, 'ignorance of physiological paternity' is
not a condition likely to characterise any human cultural groups. In
sum, Leach's position of scepticism was based on a perception of
the natural facts of procreation being *too obvious not to know.*

Leach argued that 'ignorance' in this particular context was an
oversimplified term (and he was also concerned it was a racist one).
He was consequently critical of the use of the concept of 'ignorance'
of physiological paternity to denote merely a *lack*, an *absence*, or a
deficiency of knowledge. He was reluctant to accept this use of
'ignorance' because he believed that in matters of kinship and
procreation it is never sufficient merely to point to a reported 'lack'
of knowledge without investigating *what that absence is saying.* Just
as there are many types of knowledges, so there are many types of
ignorance, he argued. Consequently, what is really at issue are
different kinds of ignorance and different kinds of truth. He wrote:

> If certain groups, such as the Trobrianders, have persuaded their
> ethnographers that they were ignorant of the facts of life, then it
> is because that 'ignorance' was for these people a kind of dogma.
> And if the ethnographer in question believed what he was told it

was because such a belief corresponded to his own private fantasy of the natural ignorance of childish savages.

(1967: 41)

Leach was particularly sensitive to the potential conflation of ignorance with primitiveness and inferiority. He wrote:

> In anthropological writing, ignorance is a term of abuse. To say that a native is *ignorant* amounts to saying he is childish, stupid, superstitious. Ignorance is the opposite of logical rationality; it is the quality which distinguishes the savage from the anthropologist.

(1967: 41, original emphasis)

Leach was elsewhere more explicitly critical of the latent evolutionary tendencies in Malinowski's work (1957: 119–39). Here as well he impugned Malinowski as an elitist who 'retained his high regard for aristocracy' throughout his life and, likewise, 'thought of "culture contact" as a kind of patronage extended by paternalistic colonial powers towards their more primitive subjects'. For Malinowski, continued Leach, 'the ignorance of the Trobrianders was a necessary element in their continuing primitiveness' (1957: 43).[10]

These claims were both highly contentious and intentionally provocative. Malinowski was not alive to answer the accusations made against him, but other anthropologists were quick to respond to Leach's remark that 'still today' there are anthropologists who 'have shown themselves willing to accept even the flimsiest evidence *for* the fact of ignorance' (1957: 46) – indeed who are 'positively *eager*' to believe in it (1957: 41). In response to Leach's *ad hominem* accusations, several anthropologists reasserted their findings of ignorance among the people they studied, and presented alternative interpretations (Schneider 1968c; Kayberry 1968; Powell 1968; Wilson 1968; Spiro 1968). Phyllis Kayberry took particular exception to the assumption that because she had believed what her informants told her she therefore thought they were 'childish, stupid and superstitious' (Kayberry 1968: 311). She also re-emphasised her findings of ignorance: 'I investigated the problem as thoroughly as possible . . . and the aborigines, despite over thirty years' contact with the whites, still had no idea of the true relation between sexual intercourse and conception' (1968: 312). Melford Spiro also responded at great length to the accusation that believing in the ignorance of a culture racist. He wrote:

[S]urely the premiss of this argument is false. . . . For, of course, ignorance is the opposite not of rationality, but of knowledge; irrationality, not ignorance, is the opposite of rationality. To be ignorant of something . . . is not necessarily to be irrational (or, for that matter, childish, stupid, superstitious, etc.). Indeed, if it were, Leach's efforts to salvage their 'rationality' by insisting that the natives are aware of physiological paternity would be in vain. For they would still be ignorant of the fact that the earth is round, that it moves around the sun, that genes are the physical basis of heredity, that man evolved from a lower primate, etc., etc.. And not only the Australians! On this premise, Europeans were irrational until the nineteenth century because they were ignorant of human evolution; until the fifteenth century because they did not believe in a heliocentric universe; and so on. In short, the premiss – ignorant = irrational – is not only semantically false, but it is culturally and historically absurd.

(Spiro 1968: 43)

Although the discussion of ignorance, what it meant or did not mean, what it can tell us and what it cannot, raised important issues of ethnographic interpretation, a key question was left out of the correspondence. This question concerned Leach's assumption that the main reason 'ignorance' is a problematic term was because the Trobrianders were not really ignorant at all. This assumption in turn depended upon Leach's claim that the 'facts of life' are too obvious not to know. It is important to ask what knowledge of the 'facts of life' Leach assumed the Trobrianders must have? What would follow from proof that the Trobrianders 'really know' that heterosexual intercourse is necessary for pregnancy to occur? From Leach's point of view it would have indicated that they were not 'ignorant' as claimed. But we would still be left with as many questions about the meaning of their knowledge as we would be otherwise about the meanings of their 'ignorance'.

The privileging of authoritative (western) scientific knowledge is clearly evident in the quotation from Spiro, in which all of the examples refer to the history of European scientific progress; to astronomy and biology in particular. What neither he nor Leach addressed directly was the issue of the relationship between 'scientific truth', as defined by modern Euro-American culture, and cultural knowledge about the natural world and the human body, as defined in other parts of the world. Implicitly the debate about ignorance assumed there was somewhere the 'real' truth (as Kayberry described it) to be known. Consistently in this debate, the truths offered by western science were presented as the 'real' truths against which other truths (or ignorance) should be defined.[11]

Whereas Malinowski addressed the question of 'virgin birth' through a functionalist argument about the nature of 'family', Leach's entire response to the question of 'virgin birth' is best understood as a structuralist argument about the nature of knowledge. Leach argued that in order to understand the professed ignorance of the Trobrianders it was first of all essential to acknowledge that 'there are different kinds of truth' (Leach 1957: 44). Secondly, one must distinguish between what is *said* and what is *meant*. Additionally it must be recognised that truths have different meanings in different contexts. This is the only means of reconciling the 'paradox' of 'why [it is that] all these people believe in something which is untrue' and the question of 'how we should interpret ethnographical statements about palpable untruth' (1957: 44). Leach argued that 'as a vulgar positivist' he could not accept the idea that 'statements of dogma start out as mistaken attempts to explain cause and effect in the world of nature' (1957: 43). Nor could he be satisfied with the 'neo-Tylorian' corollary that 'dogma persists because these mistaken ideas satisfy psychological desires' (1957: 43). Because these theories are based on hypotheses that are 'inaccessible to observation or verification' (ibid. p. 44), Leach rejected them as unscientific.

Rather, he argued, what should be recognised is '[what the dogma] "says" about the society in which it is affirmed' (1957: 43). Leach advocated this approach for several reasons:

1 it avoided the implication of ignorance which had the potential to be a derogatory classification;
2 it was a method which could be empirically and logically verified;
3 it ultimately produced more information about culture and society than other theories, and
4 it was a better theoretical basis for cross-cultural comparison.
   For example, argued Leach:
   If we put the so-called primitive beliefs alongside the sophisticated ones and treat the whole lot with equal philosophical respect we shall see that they constitute a set of variations around a common structural theme, *the metaphysical topography of the relationship between gods and men.*

(Leach 1957: 39, emphasis added)

The structuralist interpretation not only allowed for, but emphasised the extent to which beliefs about procreation articulate with a total social context of rules, institutions, rituals, belief, and, most importantly, knowledge practices. Just as 'the English marriage ritual [tells] the outside observer a great deal about the formal social relations which are being established between the various parties concerned' (1957: 40), so in the case of the Trobrianders what is *meant* is far more complex and overdetermined than what is said. 'The myth, like the rite', argued Leach, 'does not distinguish knowledge from ignorance. It establishes categories and affirms relationships' (1957: 42).

This perspective also allowed, in fact it prioritised, a greater sensitivity to *the context in which a statement was made and the importance of to whom it is addressed*. Leach's perspective allowed him to make much more useful distinctions within the ethnographic material provided by Malinowski and others because he recognised the importance of the context of informants' information. For example, Leach emphasised that in Powell's material there was a distinction made by the Trobrianders themselves between 'mission talk' and Trobriander talk about procreation (1957: 48); Powell also distinguished between '"men's talk" [which is] valid in formal situations, e.g. in matters of land ownership and the like, . . . and "women's talk" [which is] what fathers or their sisters told children [about sexuality]' (1957: 48). The very existence of these distinctions underlines the importance of the structuralist recognition that truth can simultaneously exist in multiple, and contradictory forms. What is 'true' in one context may perfectly well contradict a statement that is equally 'true' in another. However, this principle was not seen to apply to the 'truth' about paternity. Instead, argued Leach, the fact that 'there are different kinds of truth' is 'also what good Catholics say' about the Virgin Mother (1957: 44). 'Theologians who debate the doctrine of transubstantiation cannot usefully be accused of ignorance of the elementary facts of chemistry', he concluded (1957: 48). This argument avoided the question of whether some 'biological facts' are simply too obvious not to know, thus comprising a domain of 'natural fact' that is acontextual past a certain point. Instead, Leach's argument enabled him to emphasise the different ways it was possible to organise the possession of such knowledge, for example by strategically denying it.

If the structuralists are correct that in the domain of cultural meaning there are not single truths to be found, then there is no 'right' answer to the questions raised by the 'virgin birth', vulgar positivism and verifiability criteria notwithstanding. However, because the whole issue of ignorance in Leach's argument was discussed in terms of an opposition between 'the true facts' and cultural belief, this dichotomy remained unexamined. The 'virgin birth' question was again argued *in relation to* the yardstick of western cultural categories, such as 'biological facts', and this yardstick is, ironically, not very different from prejudice of social Darwinism Leach so vehemently attacked. Most certainly not from the Trobrianders' point of view. Science also has a cultural dimension, and is a form of knowledge 'as much affected by cultural elements and re-interpretations as is the case in Australia', as Malinowski himself pointed out (1937: xxxii). It is, to practice the deduction so favoured by Leach, only logical that this must be acknowledged at some level, especially in the context of anthropological discussions about reproduction and kinship. Again in this debate, the question of anthropologists own biological models was obscured beneath the mantle of objective science and 'natural fact'. Although 'truth' is contextual, 'science' is the exception, both in terms of how anthropology operates 'as a science', and in terms of how other knowledge practices are to be judged.

Spiro: the psychoanalytic interpretation of 'virgin birth'

> To say the natives transmit, generation upon generation, a conception belief in whose manifest meaning they do not believe, so that they may enunciate a structural message contained in its latent content, and in which they do believe – this can only make sense on the assumption that the latter meassge, being painful, has undergone repression, and can only be expressed by means of unconscious symbolism.
>
> (Spiro 1968: 253)

Like Leach, Melford Spiro argued the Trobrianders are not ignorant of physiological paternity: he too was concerned with how their professed ignorance should be therefore interpreted. Neither Spiro nor Leach believed the Trobrianders' ignorance could simply be understood as a lack of knowledge. Both agreed the statement of 'ignorance' indexed a structuring absence, and 'meant' something quite different from what was 'said'. In sum, neither Leach nor Spiro were prepared to accept statements of ignorance as literal truth. Their explanations for its meaning, however, divided them sharply.

In 'Virgin Birth, Parthenogenesis and Physiological Paternity: an Essay in Cultural Interpretation' (1968), Spiro argued that the beliefs of the Trobrianders regarding conception and procreation could only be understood as manifestations of the Oedipus Complex. Spiro's interpretation thus revised an argument for the universality of the Oedipus Complex, contributing to a celebrated earlier controversy between Malinowski and Ernest Jones, Sigmund Freud's industrious protégé. On the basis of the Trobriand material – including their procreation beliefs – Malinowski claimed that the Oedipus Complex was not a universal psycho-social constellation but rather a culturally specific one. He argued there was a culturally specific psycho-social constellation in the Trobriands involving a brother-sister-uncle rather than a mother-father-son constellation. He called this the Trobriand Matrilineal Complex and advocated it polemically in *Sex and Repression in Savage Society* (1927a). Conversely, Jones (1925) argued that the Trobriand case fully supported the psychoanalytic case for the Oedipus Complex as a universal feature of human psychological development (see Parsons 1964 for a detailed analysis of this controversy, and also Roheim, 1933). In his 'virgin birth' article of 1968, Spiro sided with Freud, Jones and Roheim by advocating the analytic superiority of the Oedipal model to explain Trobriand cultural constructions of procreation and conception.

Spiro argued that the question of ignorance of physiological paternity was a controversy 'for which the ethnographic facts are merely a medium of intellectual exchange'. This latter controversy was, he argued, 'theoretical and methodological in character [involving] such issues as the nature of culture, how it works, what its functions are, what explanatory variables must be attended to in attempting to interpret any of its manifestations' (1968: 253). Thus, as in the case of Leach, Spiro's argument was addressed to scientific methodology and the definition of 'truth' within anthropology, for which the 'biological facts of reproduction' served as the knowledge explicitly at issue.

Spiro's 'virgin birth' argument focused largely on the definition of ignorance used by Leach in his Henry Myers lecture of 1966. Specifically, he challenged the idea that the Trobrianders' ignorance is dogmatic, that is to say, culturally learned, and he argued this idea was unsupported by the evidence (1968: 252). What the evidence did not explain, argued Spiro, is why the structural message of the dogma of ignorance claimed by Leach could not be expressed directly. 'What function can possibly be served by enunciating this particular principle in the symbolism of conception?', he asked (1968: 253). Indeed, Leach offered no explanation for this symbolic evasion. He did not ask *why* certain messages were expressed indirectly as structural principles, nor did he address the function of statements in which people say the opposite of what they mean. He merely argued it is significant that they do so, and that all cultures have statements of this kind, particularly in relation to certain subjects such as life, death and human regeneration.

Spiro pursued this point by arguing that the central analogy of Leach's lecture, the 'virgin birth', is not a valid comparison. As the title of his article suggests, Spiro argued the correct analogy is to parthenogenesis: 'unlike the Christian dogma, the Australian belief is not about virgin births, but about non-procreative births ... the notion that conception occurs without copulation' (1968 249).[12] The analogy to 'virgin birth', he suggested, is inaccurate on several technical points. First, he argued that 'ignorance of physiological paternity' cannot possibly be the implication of the Christian dogma of immaculate conception, or 'virgin birth':

> If ... the dogma of the Virgin Birth is not held to imply that Christians are or were ignorant of physiological paternity it is because this cannot possibly be its implication. Far from claiming that the virginal conception of Jesus typifies a general norm of virginal conception, this dogma, by holding that His birth was a miracle, makes precisely the reverse claim: it denies that the norm of procreative conception applies in His case. ... [U]nlike the spirit-child belief, the Virgin Birth does not assert Jesus had no genitor, it asserts that he had no *human* genitor.
>
> (1968: 249)[13]

In fact, Leach did note that 'in its Christian context the myth of the Virgin Birth does *not* imply ignorance of the facts of physiological paternity. On the contrary, it serves to reinforce the dogma that the Virgin's child is the son of God' (1967: 42). However, Leach goes on to assert that 'the Christian doctrine of the physical-spiritual paternity of God the Father does not preclude a belief in the sociological paternity of St Joseph' (1967: 42). Noting that the Gospels of Matthew and Luke establish a pedigree for Jesus 'in the direct line of patrilineal descent from David *through Joseph*', Leach argues that the kind of belief found to be so remarkable elsewhere 'has been orthodox among Christians for about 1600 years'. This confirms his overall argument that 'the myth, like the rite, does not distinguish knowledge from ignorance. It establishes categories and affirms relationships' (1967: 42) and his core analogy that 'stories about ignorance and paternity among primitive peoples are of the same kind as stories about the virgin birth of deities in the so-called higher religions . . . we need to consider them as variations on a single structural theme' (1967: 46 fn).[14]

Spiro disagreed that the Christian dogma of the Virgin Birth expressed a sociological, rather than a biological, message. It is only the biological message, that Jesus did *not* have a human genitor, which enables the theological function of the immaculate conception to be served. Furthermore, the assertion that Jesus's relationship to Joseph was sociological rather than biological did not 'establish categories and affirm relationships' within Christianity: it was instead a point of considerably theological controversy and debate. On the one hand, Spiro argues, as Saviour Jesus cannot have a human pedigree (because he is God). On the other hand, as Christ, He must have had a human genitor to be a direct descendent of David. Hence, 'the very criterion by which [the doctrine of the Virgin Birth] established the claim that Jesus is Saviour disqualified Him from the claim that He is Messiah' (1968: 252). It should be added, of course, that the doctrine of the Virgin Birth of Jesus is precisely what distinguishes Judaism (for whom Jesus was not the son of God, but an influential prophet) from Christianity (within which his divinity is the primary article of faith). However, since Jesus is both Messiah, and Christ the Saviour within Christendom, Spiro's point that 'nothing could be more absurd than the suggestion that the function of Jesus' Davidic genealogy (let alone the Virgin Birth) is to affirm the structural principle [of sociological paternity]', or, as Leach also argued, of patrilateral filiation, remains valid.

Even if, Spiro argued, sociological paternity *were* affirmed by the doctrine of the Virgin Birth, this still raises the question of why, if genitorship is known, patership is selected as the basis on for paternity and patrilateral filiation, as Leach suggests? There is no necessary correlation between knowledge or ignorance of physiological paternity and the principle of patrilateral filiation, Spiro claimed (1968: 255). This left the question, still, of 'what could possibly be the motive for rejecting genitorship as the basis for fatherhood' (1968: 254), since, as both Spiro and Leach assumed, it must be known, and therefore not be *absent* but for some reason *rejected*.

Spiro offers an alternative, functionalist, explanation to those of either Leach or Malinowski. He argued that statements which have to be expressed indirectly, and in which people say the opposite of what they know to be true, are evidence of repression:

> To say the natives transmit, generation upon generation, a conception belief in whose manifest meaning they do not believe, so that they may enunciate a structural message contained in its latent content, and in which they do believe – this can only make sense on the assumption that the latter message, being painful, has undergone repression, and can only be expressed by means of unconscious symbolism.
>
> (1968: 253)

On the basis of this argument, Spiro also challenged Leach's rejection of Malinowski's findings of ignorance among the Trobrianders. The idea of repression, and the theory of the unconscious on which it depends, allowed Spiro to argue that the Trobrianders were *both ignorant and knowing simultaneously*: they were consciously ignorant but unconsciously knowing. Like Jones, Spiro believed that the Trobrianders were not 'ignorant' as a result of the *absence* of biological knowledge, but because they had *denied and repressed* it. Therefore their procreation beliefs should not be interpreted as existing *in default* of the 'true facts' but rather *in lieu* of them.

This interpretation led Spiro directly to the Oedipal Complex as an explanation for repression. In his later monograph on the subject, *Oedipus in the Trobriands* (1984), Spiro presented an extended argument for this interpretation in order to defend his claim that the Trobrianders can no longer stand as the test case for rejecting the universality of the Oedipus Complex. To the contrary, Spiro argued, the fact of physiological paternity is repressed to such an extent by the Trobrianders that the Oedipus Complex must be even stronger in their culture than it is in Euro-American context.

The elaboration of his 'virgin birth' article in *Oedipus in the Trobriands* contains Spiro's extended argument along these lines. Malinowski's ethnographic data form the basis for many of his conclusions, and particular attention is given to Trobriand beliefs about procreation. Using these data, Spiro claims that the absence of the father in Trobriand myths, dreams and reproductive beliefs is an act of 'symbolic patricide' by Trobriand males (1984: 65). It is the expression of 'patricidal wishes' aroused by the son's (Spiro does not discuss daughters) 'painful recognition' that 'his father is [his] genitor' and therefore that his 'father enjoys sexual possession of [his] mother whom he himself has desired', thus 'remind[ing] him that she, in turn, has betrayed him by preferring [his] father to him' (1984: 65). The repression occurs because 'the awareness of parental intercourse, *according at least to Oedipal theory*, is always painful to the child for those reasons' (1984: 65, emphasis added). Furthermore, he argues, 'the recognition that the father is genitor is painful for the son because . . . it reminds him that his very existence was brought about by that hated sexual relationship that the father has with the mother' (1984: 66). He concludes that 'unable to cope in a realistic fashion with the emotional pain or threat that is aroused by their recognition of the reproductive role of the father, [Trobriand males] attempt to cope instead in a magical fashion – by eliminating the father as genitor and putting another genitor, a spirit-child, in his place' (1984: 64).[15] According to Spiro, this explains why the Trobrianders do not believe sexual intercourse causes pregnancy, and he suggests that the spirit-child theory allows the Trobriand male child to imagine that *he is his own genitor*, corresponding to a keenly desired masculine fantasy of omnipotence (1984: 68).

It is not within the scope of this discussion to reproduce the full spectrum of psychoanalytic arguments offered in defence of Spiro's claims, although it is worth noting that they depart considerably from the classic psycho-analytic arguments put forward by either Sigmund Freud or Ernest Jones. Neither is it undertaken here to explore fully Spiro's use of Trobriand ethnographic data to support his claims (see Weiner 1985 for clarification on this point). Rather, what is significant here is his treatment of 'biological facts'. Although Spiro's theory offers hypothetical explanations for many aspects of the Trobrianders' beliefs about procreation that were left unresolved by Malinowski and Leach, he leaves unanswered the central question of the presumed self-evidentness of 'the facts of life'. Spiro is identical to Leach in this respect: he simply assumes that the recognition of certain biological 'truths' is a given – *so obvious it needs no explanation.* Indeed it is the utter impossibility of ignorance that is the premise of both arguments, in a debate singularly characterised by an apparent fury to leave no first premises unscathed.

Like the structuralism of Leach, the functionalism of Malinowski, and the evolutionism of nineteenth-century social theorists, Spiro's psychoanalytic model uncritically relies upon the presumed self-evidentness of the 'biological facts' of reproduction, once again revealing how essential is their givenness to social theory. Across all of these analytical approaches, and across several generations of theoretical debate, the consistency with which an unchanging model of biological reproduction structures central premises of inquiry, and remains itself invisible even to rudimentary questioning, emerges as a cultural fact of some importance in its own right.

Consequent upon the presumption of the structuring importance of 'the facts of life' as they are defined by western biological science (the facts that are consistently deemed 'too obvious not to know') are enormous theoretical consequences, the scope of which under-scores the breadth of territory rendered unexaminable by their status as a given.[16] The production of sexual difference, the maintenance of heterosexuality, the operations of an *a priori* domain of 'natural fact', the presumption of a reproductive telos at the base of social organisation, and the contradictions all of these forms of cultural reproduction must entail, all consistently evade critical *recognition* (not to mention discussion) as a result of being so taken-for-granted they remain invisible. Finally, it must be noted that these features comprising the invisible givens of a century of anthropological debate addressing the significance of beliefs about conception and procreation, on which so much else was clearly founded, can be directly traced to the post-Darwinian worldview of Euro-American anthropology. It is Darwin's 'plot', in both its narrative and carto-graphic senses, which precisely foregrounded the importance of nature-as-consanguinity (the 'tree of life' analogy through which Darwin unified nature as a 'system').[16] In turn, this must be structured by a reproductive telos of cumulative change, which centrally depends upon binary sexual difference, or, as Darwin put it, 'sexual selection'. Just as Spiro's argument is unashamedly concerned exclusively to explicate 'the descent of man' and its psychic permuta-tions in the form of the Oedipus complex, so he is also willing to position this dynamic at the core of a universal, 'scientific' ex-planation of culture. In addressing the question of male ignorance so thoroughly, for it is primarily the ignorance of the male in relation to his own paternity with which the debates from the 1860s to the 1960s were concerned, it is tempting to speculate upon the operations of denial, exclusion and wish-fulfilment among the contestants as a more convincing exemplification of Oedipal psychic conflict than is offered by Spiro for the Trobrianders.

Schneider: biology as a symbolic system

> These biological facts . . . have as one of their aspects a symbolic quality, which means that they represent something other than what they are, over and above and in addition to their existence as biological facts.
>
> (Schneider 1968b: 116)

Writing as a correspondent to *Man* in response to Spiro's 'virgin birth' article, David Schneider recounted an episode from his fieldwork among the Yapese. Like the Trobrianders, Schneider's informants emphatically denied any causal relation between heterosexual intercourse and pregnancy. He was thus 'unnerved' by a conversation with four men he discovered removing the testicles from a small pig. 'Could a sow ever get pregnant from such a boar?' he asked 'slyly'. 'Not from that one!', the men replied, explaining that a boar whose testicles had not been removed would be necessary to impregnate a sow. 'Castrate the pig and he grows larger than if he is not castrated', Schneider repeated. 'Right!' the men replied. 'But a castrated pig cannot make a sow pregnant', he continued. 'Right!' they affirmed. 'But . . . everyone has been telling me that coitus does not make women pregnant' he persisted. 'That is correct', the men replied, puzzled by Schneider's apparent confusion. He explained:

> We did not understand one another. I had presented them, I felt, with logically inconsistent statements that fairly cried out for some explanation. They could not see what my problem was since they had provided me with the full array of necessary, correct facts and to them there was no problem. So we kept at it until I again put the contradiction to them; if you castrate a pig he cannot get a sow pregnant. Surely that proved that copulation causes pregnancy! But suddenly one man saw what my problem was, for he put it plainly and emphatically: "But people are not pigs!" Once that point was made, the rest followed in happy, logical order. I had obviously assumed that biological processes opererated for all animals, and had included man among them. But they had assumed that no one but a fool would equate people with pigs.
>
> (1968c: 127–8)

As this account suggests, Schneider's importance to the 'virgin birth' debates, and to the attempt to grapple with the relationship of the 'biological facts' of human reproduction to anthropological explanation, derives from his attempt to separate the 'facts' of biological reproduction as scientific truth, from their operation as forms of cultural knowledge. Although this perspective replaces the dichotomy of 'natural' and social facts with that between biology as science and science as culture, it is a move that opened up an important space for much later work on kinship and gender, as the final section of this chapter makes clear. In his contribution to the 'virgin birth' debates, Schneider made the simple point that it is not a universally shared assumption that the making of new persons is commensurate with the littering of pigs. By reversing the 'problem' of ignorance to foreground his own 'hidden' assumptions, Schneider revealed his own 'unnerving' encounter with a perfectly 'obvious' logic (that 'people are not pigs'). 'Obvious' though this distinction may be, when stated so 'plainly and emphatically', it none the less unseats the core analogy of the Darwinian model of nature, that people are not only 'like', but consanguinous with and descended from animals.

In *American Kinship: a cultural account*, published in the same year as his 'virgin birth' correspondence (1968b), Schneider discussed this issue in greater depth, and closer to home. His approach was theoretically and methodologically distinctive, in so far as it could be described as an ethnography of cultural constructions of the natural. Much of Schneider's early work concerned the relationship between natural and social facts in kinship theory (Schneider 1964, 1965, 1968a, b and c, 1972). He provided what remains one of the definitive treatments of this longstanding opposition in his later volume *A Critique of the Study of Kinship*, published in 1984, which is discussed at greater length in the final section. His ethnographic monograph on American kinship anticipates, though it also exemplifies, his later argument that despite superficial modifications, the implicit frame of reference informing the analysis of kinship systems from Morgan to the present has remained 'the biological facts' of sexual reproduction. He argued it is the hegemonic status of biological science in Euro-American anthropology which continues to bias kinship research towards an assumption of genetic ('natural') relatedness as logically prior to any other system, and as the implicit material base for kinship superstructures. Just as religion has been defined as categories relating to the supernatural, he argued, so kinship has been defined as categories relating to the natural. 'I do not assume', he stated, 'that this domain is defined *a priori* by the biogenetic premises of the genealogically defined grid' (1972: 37).

Schneider's interpretive/symbolic approach to the meanings of American kinship categories diverged from the view that the fundamental units of kinship are genetic by taking *the symbols of kinship themselves* as the objects of study. By so doing, he demonstrated how concepts of procreation in American culture illuminate certain other basic formal problems such as the separation of public and private spheres, the opposition between love and money, and the sexual division of labour. He thus situated the cultural system of kinship, based on the *symbolism* of biology and nature, within a total social context of American beliefs, institutions and practices across a wide variety of domains.

According to Schneider's analysis, American kinship can be described as a dominant cultural logic, decipherable in terms of the operation of core symbols, oppositions and dictates. Theoretically, his aim was to elucidate the independent workings of culture as a distinct level of the social order.[17] As such, his analysis of American kinship as a cultural system exemplified a symbolic anthropological approach to culture. In his now classic monograph on American kinship (1968b), just over 100 pages in length, he argued that coitus is the central symbol in the 'symbolic universe' of American kinship. It is through heterosexual reproduction that children are connected to their parents by 'shared biogenetic substance' which symbolises 'diffuse, enduring solidarity', represented in the vernacular as 'blood ties' (1968b: 34–9). Coitus is the symbol naturalising the unity of the conjugal and procreative function, affirmed by progeny who are equally related to both the mother's and the father's 'sides'. 'Nature' is the dominant idiom of this cultural system:

> The family is formed according to the laws of nature and it lives by rules which are regarded by Americans as self-evidently natural. . . . The fact of nature on which the cultural construct of of the family is based is . . . that of sexual intercourse. This figure provides all of the cultural symbols of American kinship. Sexual intercourse is a natural act with natural consequences according to its cultural definition.
>
> (1968b: 34–9)

The 'natural' act of coitus between two people who are biogenetically unrelated but legally married provides the symbolic link between the order of nature (relations of blood) and the order of law (relations through marriage, e.g. 'in-laws'). These are the two primary symbolic domains of American kinship, conjoined by natural fact of coitus which is thus the 'core symbol' within the American kinship 'universe'.

However, within the functional and 'obvious' logic of this dominant code of conduct are also significant sources of tension and contradiction. Schneider pointed out some of these:

> The relationship between man and nature in American culture is an active one. . . . Man's place is to dominate nature, to control it, to use nature's powers for his own ends. . . . In American culture man's fate is seen as one which follows the injunction Master Nature!
>
> But at home things are different. Where kinship and the family are concerned, American culture appears to turn things topsy-turvy. . . . What is out there in Nature, say the definitions of American culture, is what kinship is. . . . To be otherwise is unnatural, artificial, contrary to nature.
>
> (1968b: 107)

Schneider discusses sexual intercourse as a case in point. On the one hand, it is 'natural', it is 'what animals do'. On the other hand, it is also morally circumscribed in that it must be confined to the context of marriage, be performed genital to genital, occur in private, not be discussed publicly, etc. It is both 'natural' and an improvement upon 'nature' at the same time.

Schneider rationalised this contradiction by arguing that since Americans believe man is 'a special part' of nature, due to his 'capacity for reason', he is at once part of nature and above its dictates. However, this explanation merely accounted for how Americans rationalise the contradictions within their own belief systems. It did not address the question of what this contradiction reveals about the operations of 'dominant' symbolic systems, or the extent to which they can, as Schneider proposed, be described as coherent.

A useful historical perspective on this problem is provided by Collier, Rosaldo and Yanagisako in their social-historical account of the family and anthropological approaches to it. In 'Is there a Family' (1982), the authors note a number of significant changes in the evolution of the modern nuclear family. As recently as the Victorian era, they point out, the idea of the family as a 'natural' institution would have been considered barbaric. The idea of unrestricted sexual intercourse as the basis of kinship systems was precisely the notion that led Morgan and other evolutionists to postulate the existence of primitive promiscuity and group marriage. If sexual intercourse was the 'natural' basis for kinship, argued these early theorists, then 'man's' 'natural' (i.e. sexual) urges would inevitably lead to promiscuity and illegitimacy thereby precluding the formation of monogamous marriage or nuclear family groups. Rather than being founded on a 'natural' basis, the Victorians believed the family to be founded on a *moral* one. The idea that they lived in families because it was 'natural' would have been unacceptable – if not nonsensical – within the Victorian worldview. The significance of the family as a moral institution was precisely that it was *not* natural, not 'what animals do', or, for that matter, what primitive savages did, as far as the Victorians were concerned. That the family had a moral rather than a 'natural' basis signified to Victorian society that its family structure was a cultural achievement, not a 'natural fact'.

It is clear from Schneider's analysis of American kinship beliefs, although he did not underscore it himself, that there are at least three different 'natures' involved in defining what is 'natural': as *biology* ('shared biogenetic substance'); as *what animals do* ('Americans see a pair of wolves with their cubs in their cave as a family' (1968b: 109)); and as *human nature* (man is a 'special part' of nature). There are also many different 'natures' in terms of what they are defined in opposition to. 'Unnatural', 'artifical', 'cultural', 'human', 'reason', 'civilized', 'superior' and 'abnormal' all appeared in Schneider's account as the opposite of 'natural'. As Raymond Williams has argued, '*Nature* is perhaps the most complex word in the [English] language' and 'any full history of the uses of *nature* would be a history of a large part of human thought' (1981: 219–21).

It was for all of these reasons somewhat unsatisfactory that alongside his suggestive discussion of the symbolic importance of ideas of 'nature' to American kinship as a cultural system, Schneider sought to emphasise the coherence of nature/biology as a symbolic idiom for American kinship, and to preserve a separate scientific definition of natural/biological 'facts' as scientific. He was both explicit and unequivocal in his effort to retain a strict separation between 'biological facts' as scientific truth and these same 'facts' as cultural symbols. He wrote:

The biological prerequisites for human existence exist and remain. The child . . . does not come into being except by the fertilized egg . . . These are the biological facts. They are facts of life and facts of nature.

(1968b: 116)

Schneider underscored this distinction clearly: 'So much of kinship and family in American culture is defined as being nature itself, required by nature, or directly determined by nature that it is quite difficult . . . for Americans to see this as a set of cultural constructs *and not the biological facts themselves*' (1968b: 116, emphasis added). For Schneider, the important point was that the 'real', 'true', 'facts' of biological science *also* have a cultural function. He explained:

These biological facts . . . have *as one of their aspects* a symbolic quality, which means that they represent something *other than what they are*, over and above and *in addition to* their existence as biological facts.

(1968b: 116, emphasis added)

Thus, although his work represented an important effort to explore the symbolic dimension of natural facts, it explicitly preserved the same separation between culture and biology he started with. On the one hand, Schneider was arguing that there is no such thing as a biological fact *per se* in American kinship systems – there are only cultural interpretations of them. On the other hand, he was also arguing that there *are* 'natural facts' within science which are true and which are separate from the cultural constructions of them. This required that 'biological facts' lead a separate existence in the laboratory, protected by the authoritative discourses of natural science from the rest of culture. But, if there are two different dimensions of 'biological fact' – the scientific one and the symbolic one – then must not there exist a relationship between the two? If 'biology' persists as a separate, unassailable domain of knowledge, then what is its status in relation to the rest of culture? Or is it acultural? Is this not an argument that biology *must be* logically prior to cultural meaning?

Part of the problem lies in the term 'biology' itself, which refers both to physical phenomena, such as the human body, as in 'the biology of the human species', and to *the study of* such phenomena, as in 'I failed human biology as a graduate student'. There is, significantly, no such corollary isomorphism for 'sociology', which has as its object 'society'. The conflation of the object to be known with the discipline of its observation and description terminological performs the collapsing of knowledge with its object distinctive of modern western scientific ways of knowing. Indeed, that is the definitively scientific 'collapse': that objective knowledge in the sciences is so transparent it is isomorphic with the reality it describes, a premise which revealingly does not hold true for 'sciences' such as anthropology.

But, as Schneider's work on American kinship demonstrated, the status of the biological in social theory has had a kind of Teflon protection: near as the critique might come to sticking, it was always sliding off at the penultimate moment, unable to adhere. Hence, despite arguing that biology could be seen to operate as a 'folk theory' of kinship in the context of American culture, achieving full-blown symbolic elaboration, to the point of wildly convoluted 'dictates' about where the determinism of nature/biology was to be followed, these 'facts' emerge with untarnished credentials as authoritative scientific knowledge none the less.

Of course, as every Euro-American now knows, not even Teflon lasts forever, and these are precisely the questions Schneider later turned to in his reassessment of the history of anthropological accounts of kinship in 1984. Mounting a critique of the persistent separation of 'natural' and social facts in the study of kinship, for which his own earlier work served as an exemplary case, he argues that kinship theory ultimately reveals more about the influence of folk European categories in the history of social science than it does about the 'simple societies' for whom it has long been assumed to be a principle feature of social organisation. Anticipating the wave of auto-critique that swept through anthropology in the mid-1980s, *A Critique of the Study of Kinship* concluded that the core features defining the study of kinship since its inception are insupportable, unworkable and illegitimate.

This powerful argument began to pave the way for a different approach to kinship, and for its analysis *as* a 'folk European theory' not only in relation to its historical importance to European social theory, but ethnographically, as has recently begun to be demonstrated (Edwards *et al.* 1993; Ginsburg 1989; Hayden 1995; Lewin 1993; Ragone 1994; Weston 1991). It is no coincidence that both Schneider's early volume on American kinship, and his later archaeology of kinship knowledge in *Critique* . . . have become central reference points in the study of lesbian and gay kinship and kinship in the context of new reproductive technologies: two of the rapidly expanding sites in which 'kinship' is once again being reinvented – this time for use where it is arguably most revealing, in the Euro-American cultures where it had its own beginnings.

Two of the Schneiderian precepts which have become most centrally debated in these and other studies are the coherence of 'the natural' as a cultural 'order', and consequently the 'coherence' of symbolic systems as 'cultural logics' at all (see especially Strathern 1992a). The Schneiderian model of 'a cultural system' can be glossed as one of 'dominant ideology' in more political terms. It is an anthropological model of culture which has much in common with what might be described in more contemporary terms as 'the hegemonic discourse'. However, both the concept of hegemony, drawn from Gramsci, and the model of discourse drawn from Foucault, emphasise the instability, contradictoriness and inbuilt sources of tension characteristic of 'dominant' cultural systems. In terms of ideology, both of these points, and the additional instability at the level of subjectivity and identity emphasised within psycho-analysis, have been argued by Stuart Hall to comprise an important shift away from more rationalist models of 'dominant cultural logic'.[18]

One of the advantages of combining anthropological and cultural studies is the greater range of explanatory models their admixture can produce, and also the greater precision available at the level of cultural theory derivative of their being put into conversation with one another. Ideas of the natural comprise one of the most important 'cultural logics' that more recent theorists of kinship and gender have sought to analyse. For the study of both Englishness and Americanness, this idiom is essential. But it is important to specify what is meant by a 'cultural logic' of the natural. Developing models with which to theorise both the levels of coherence, and of contradictory tensions, within the domain of the natural constitutes an ongoing and expanding area of contemporary social theory. Schneider's work has continued to influence debates about kinship, gender and sexuality for precisely this reason, much as his work also foregrounds many of the shortcomings these later debates have sought to overcome.

Weiner: redefining reproduction

I analyze reproduction not as a biological construct, but as a cultural concept in which the basic process for reproducing human beings, social relations, cosmological phenomena, and material resources are culturally defined and structurally interconnected.

(Weiner 1978: 183)

Among the many features of Trobriand society reanalysed by Annette Weiner in the 1970s in contrast to the approaches developed by Malinowski half a century before was the significance of conception beliefs to principles of social organisation (1976). Her approach to reproduction was both influenced by and a major contribution to the ongoing work of feminist anthropologists in the 1970s which aimed not only to uncover the roles of women cross-culturally, but to redefine the paradigms in anthropology resultant from their previous exclusion (see especially Weiner 1995). Towards this end, Weiner provided some of the most important ethnographic and theoretical contributions to redefinitions of core theoretical concerns with kinship, gender and exchange (1978, 1979, 1995). Her model of reproduction was central to this effort.

Weiner's analysis of kinship and reproduction avoided the pitfall of dichotomising culture and biology by means of a theoretical readjustment so simple and straightforward it is revealing in itself that it was so completely overlooked until the 1970s. Weiner simply argued that the reproduction of Trobrianders is not a biological process but a cultural achievement. A 'purely' biological process is simply insufficient to produce a Trobriander. This is a radical extension of Malinowski's argument that:

> The ideas and institutions which control conception, pregnancy and birth show that these cannot be regarded by the anthropologist as mere physiological facts, but as facts deeply modified by culture and social organisation.
>
> (Malinowski 1962: 140)

Weiner substantially enlarged upon and documented Malinowski's argument that the meaning of Trobriand procreation beliefs must be understood in relation to their total social context. She extended this context to include *transgenerational time* as part of the process of reproduction. Thus, reproduction is analysed not only in terms of the individual life-cycle, starting with the death of an ancestor who returns as a spirit-child, but in terms of interconnecting life-cycles over time, and the longterm reproduction and maintenance of the matrilineage.

Because biological reproduction is only sufficient to produce a biological human being, but not a Trobriander, Weiner's model of reproduction encompassed much more than 'physiological facts'. Reproduction, she argued, is a process among the Trobrianders which ties together sociological, cosmological, material and physical dimensions of their culture. It is a process that involves an extensive network of kinship ties which are mobilised to contribute to the growth of the child in both cultural and physical terms (see Weiner 1988). Many different kinds of social relationships are called upon to contribute to the production of a new human being, including sexual relationships, exchange relationships, affinal relationships, conjugal relationships, and relationships among clan members Most importantly, she demonstrated that the reproduction of *dala* identity, of the matrilineage, is 'an integral and complementary part of the processes of human reproduction and the reproduction of social relations' (1979: 329). This is because cultural identity, which is the crucial difference between a Trobriander and a mere biological human, is primarily achieved through kinship, through the establishment of a person's position in relation to their ancestry, their matrilineage, their clan, their parents and their siblings. In sum, the establishment of kin ties is the establishment not only of cultural identity but of *humanity* among the Trobrianders.

In contrast to the Trobriand model, it is biology that provides dominant Euro-American definitions of life and death, the meanings of pregnancy and birth, and the social relationships defined as kinship. This has had a significant impact on the theorisation of reproduction, in Weiner's view:

> Traditionally, reproduction has been viewed in its biological context only. In our own society, we attach little public value to the fact of reproduction, and we forget that a similar view may not be universally shared. In other societies, the *cultural* domain of reproduction may be the very basis ... through which social and cosmological concerns are integrated.
>
> (Weiner 1978: 175)

Weiner's descriptions of conception, pregnancy and the early nurturing of the young child among the Trobrianders demonstrated well the significance of this claim. Conception itself is believed to be caused by the entry of the ancestral spirit into the woman's body. It is the combination of the woman's blood and the ancestral spirit (*sibububula*) which form the fetus and give it its matrilineal identity (1988: 55). Even before the child is born, both men and women play an integral role in assisting its growth, as the Trobrianders believe that frequent sexual intercourse following conception helps to feed the child (1988: 61). This ties the child not only to its mother's matrilineage but to its father's matrilineage as well, which ties are publicly reaffirmed and reciprocated throughout the duration of the child's life.

Weiner stressed the importance of the belief in 'virgin birth' in delineating the different contributions made by women and men to the production of children. '[U]nderlying the . . . use of "virgin birth" is the belief that men and women contribute differently to conception and the growth of the fetus' (1976: 12). A man's procreative role in the birth of the child is considered essential not only for its physical growth but for its social identity as well. 'A child without a father, even though it may be well taken care of by its mother and matrilineal kin is socially disadvantaged. . . . To be "fatherless" is to be denied an essential part of one's self' (1976: 63). This is not merely a product of convention. It is the child's own interests which are at stake, for being fatherless means that half of the kinship ties the child would have had available for its own social potential are lost.

The physical contributions to the child's body from both the mother and the father are affirmed at its birth. The child is given a name by the mother from her own matrilineage which emphasizes the central idea in Trobriand conception beliefs that *matrikin are of the same body*. This does not imply the mother is the genetrix, however, for it is the ancestor which supplies the generative agency. The child is believed physically to resemble its father. Whereas this paternal resemblance has been interpreted by many participants in the 'virgin birth' debates as a substitute or incomplete recognition of the father's 'actual', e.g. biological, contribution to the child, Weiner demonstrates that this principle is fully consistent with the father's *social* role in nurturing his child.

Thus, although both the mother and the father make essential contributions to the child, they are distinctive, and *neither* contribution relies on a notion of a generative parental contribution of shared substance. Unlike the western model of procreation based on the sciences of biology and genetics, in which both parents are believed to make identical generative contributions of shared bodily substance to the formation of the child (twenty-three chromosomes each), the Trobriander's belief in qualitatively different parental contributions reflects their emphasis upon qualitatively different parental roles, *neither of which depend upon the notion of gener-ativity.*[19] As a member of the same matrilineal group, the child has inalienable rights to its mother's name and other property from her matrilineage. Because the child has only use rights to its father's name and matrilineal property, the father's gifts to his children have a different importance (1976: 60).

Contrary to Spiro's assertions, Weiner observed that both mothers and fathers lavish much affection on the young.

> Mothers nurse their infants on demand, never allowing them to cry if hungry. Men with young children walk around the village holding a baby or toddler straddled on their hips, often with another child in tow. Even very old men who stay in the village while everyone else is working in the gardens, look after their grandchildren in this way.
>
> (1976: 64)

A father feeds his child even while it is still nursing and once a child is weaned it sleeps with its father (1976: 65). A father is also responsible for the physical beauty of his children, which requires special beauty magic and shell decorations. One of the first decorations a father may provide for his child is a necklace of *Chama* discs, which are made out of the same material as the *kula* shells. This necklace signifies the father's economic responsibility for the child and his role as a provider. It also connects the child to the father's trading networks and thus extends the network of adults contributing to its welfare. 'When a child wears a necklace its value is attached to the child not only as a representation of the child's father's political worth, but as a statement of the political potential of the child as well' (1976: 67).

The extent to which reproduction in the Trobriand Islands is situated in a nexus of reciprocal obligations and exchange is thus firmly established by early infancy. The 'biological' processes involved in conception are themselves implicated in these networks and it is the work of many other people who build and maintain the relationships that give the child a social identity as well as bodily form. This view of reproduction as inseparable from the total social context in which the child's identity is given meaning and value demonstrates the limitations of the cellular model of conception against which the Trobriander's views of procreation have long been pointlessly compared. In sum, Weiner's model of reproduction is one that fully acknowledges the difference between a conceptus and a Trobriander.

By analysing reproduction in this manner, Weiner also introduced an important model for the study of kinship and gender. Once biological reproduction is no longer 'the axis on which all else turns', it is clear that 'the issues are . . . more complex'. The roles of women are no longer confined to being 'reproductive agents (and usually nothing more)' and the roles of men no longer those of 'non-reproductive agents (and everything else)' (1978: 328). In this view of reproduction, physical and cultural 'facts' are inextricable from one another and interdependent – indeed co-constutitive. Biological reproduction is not simply a 'fact of life', 'after' which cultural forms are constructed. Rather it is the total process of cultural regeneration in which human regeneration is explicitly embedded, or 'contained', and it is through this enframement that it derives its meaning, value and importance.

The value of Weiner's model is supported by evidence from Schneider concerning the conception beliefs of the Yapese, which underwent transformation from the time of his fieldwork in 1947–8 to encompass the 'western' view of conception twenty years later. The newly received model of conception was that 'the man plants a seed in the woman and the woman is like a garden', true to the Aristotelian and Judaeo-Christian roots of the western 'biological' view. Yet, as Schneider notes, according to 'the new conception of conception . . . the spirit *marialang* controls this process, just as it always did, and the process of conception cannot take place without the spirit's approval and active help'. Hence, 'the introduction of the acknowledgement of the role of coitus in conception has changed nothing . . . it is the care and protection of the seed by the woman and the *performance* of the woman as a good woman which produces the child' (1984: 73). He continues, 'even when coitus is recognized as a factor in conception it is not taken to "mean" anything radically new or different . . . It is simply not culturally significant . . . the Yapese definition . . . remains radically different from the European cultural conception of reproduction' (1984: 73).

Here, as in Weiner's argument, the scientific view of the 'true' facts of reproduction is simply irrelevant, *even when it is explicitly held*. As Scheffler and Lounsbury stated the matter bluntly in 1971:

Most well documented folk theories of human reproduction hold that sexual intercourse is a necessary part of the process, not merely that virgins cannot conceive. It is not always held to be sufficient for conception or pregnancy because, for example, it is widely appreciated that not all acts of sexual intercourse result in pregnancy. To account for this fact many folk theories hold that other-than-human or "supernatural" agencies may also play a part. According to some theories ... certain spiritual entities *activate* the foetus which itself results from events or processes associated with sexual intercourse.

(Scheffler and Lounsbury 1971: 38)

Indeed, the precise mechanisms accounting for the vicissitudes of conception have only become increasingly unclear in the context of more detailed scientific knowledge occasioning the removal of conception from the womb by late-twentieth century scientific researchers, first achieved in Britain in 1978. Weiner's suggestion, published in the same year, that 'in our own society, we attach little public value to the fact of reproduction', whereas in other societies 'reproduction may be the very basis ... through which social and cosmological concerns are integrated' (1978: 175) acquires a new 'spin' in such a context. In England too, 'it is widely appreciated that not all acts of sexual intercourse result in pregnancy'. To account for this fact, biological science provides an increasing amount of information, which, as later chapters discuss in depth, often sheds little light on why the conceptus fails to 'activate'. The study of the process of 'activation' in embryonic development is a science which dates back to Aristotle, and has remained epistemologically central to the life sciences since the birth of modern embryology. Like the study of evolution, which is also keyed to questions about origins and development, embryology and reproductive biology continue to provide powerful narrative accounts 'through which social and cosmological concerns are integrated'. It is for this reason reproduction, the value of life itself, and ideas of the natural comprise powerful domains of moral importance and cultural values in contemporary Euro-American society.

Weiner's recognition of the extent to which models of biological reproduction recapitulate models of cultural reproduction takes on added importance in the context of the contemporary effort to extend Schneider's account of 'biology as a cultural system'. In the context of projects such as the effort to map the human genome, for example, it is arguable a very explicit language of 'transcendence' is operative, for example in the popular media denominations of the Genome project as 'man's second creation' or as the quest to unlock 'the secret of life', in the form of science's 'Holy Grail'. The transcendent value of scientific rationality is often most evident precisely at the point of its encounter with life-processes, and this has long been the case.

An implication of Schneider's syncretic Yapese conception story is not only that possession of the 'true facts' is compatible with pre-exisiting models of spirit-children, but that the 'true facts' are of limited value even to those for whom they are the *only* explanatory model. As Scheffler and Lounsbury point out, it is widely, if not universally, recognised that not all acts of sexual intercourse result in pregnancy. With the growing number of couples for whom coitus *never* results in pregnancy, or for whom even conception and implantation do not result in pregnancy, the usefulness of the 'biological model' is also in question. It is increasingly the case, for a growing number of people, that 'the biological facts' explain very little indeed.

This presents an odd paradox in relation to the 'facts of life' in the Euro-American tradition which 'invented' them as such. On the one hand, as 'biological facts', these processes are seen to embody the mysteries and splendour of life itself, its great and awesome power, and its manifold diversity. In the history of scientific descriptions of 'life' is a long record of just such 'transcendental' and worshipful accounts of its elusive mystery and importance (Franklin 1995b).

At the very same time, the 'facts of life' in their strictly biological sense can be seen to explain less and less, if anything at all, in the context of failure to conceive. As later chapters demonstrate in some detail, years of pursuing the most technologically and scientifically advanced scrutiny of conceptive failure may yield enormous amounts of biological information which translate into absolutely zero knowledge. 'Unexplained' infertility is not an unusual diagnosis: it is the outcome of approximately a third of all infertility investigations. Even when a 'cause' is found, it may not entirely explain very much at all. For that matter, the most exact and complete of diagnostic information will not explain why a particular form of conceptive failure happened to affect a particular person, or couple.

The 'biological facts' of reproduction, in the Euro-American context to which they are 'native folk models', thus can be seen to explain 'everything and nothing'. At their most exalted pitch, and especially from the post-Darwinian perspective, 'life's progression' explains everything else, as the prominent natural scientist Richard

Dawkins argues in his well-known writings on the subject. All of human culture and society, all of human history and politics, and even humans themselves are mere repositories for the reproduction of genes, in his view (1976, 1986, 1995). On the other hand, for the population described in Chapters 3, 4 and 5, the biological facts of conception often explain nothing at all. And there are many variations on these two perspectives in between.

Weiner's insights thus carry important implications even for the societies she describes as attaching 'little public value to the fact of reproduction' (1978: 175). From a different perspective, British, European and American cultures have long attached quite considerable public value to the fact of reproduction, but this may have been 'hidden' in part by the supposed self-evidentness of 'the facts of life'. This and other perpsectives on the 'facts of life', which bring us up to date with more recent accounts of their significance to anthropology, are discussed in the following section, with which this chapter concludes.

AFTER VIRGIN BIRTH

So far in this chapter, several contributions to the 'virgin birth' debate have been presented to foreground the role of the 'biological facts of human reproduction' as a given within this historic controversy. As has been illustrated, Malinowski relied on a distinction between 'natural and social facts' which enabled him to establish an analytical realm of 'fact' consistent with indigenous conception theories. However, this was a frame within a frame: stepping back into the position of scientific observer, Malinowski repositioned 'social facts' within a wider analysis in which they are not literal, but functional, assertions. Similarly, Leach embraced the contextual diversity of facts, arguing that structural patterns of meaning unite the various forms of strategic disingenuousness that are encountered cross-culturally. The key to this pattern is the categorical imperative: for Leach, as for Lévi-Strauss, cultural meaning expresses an implicit order which can be unlocked at a deep structural level. Spiro's view is not dissimilar, in that he too sought an explanation for statements in which people say the opposite of what they know to be true. In his functionalist account of the operations of repression and sublimation, he again offered a truth that is accessible to the analyst alone.

Both Weiner and Schneider move towards explicit recognition of the role of biological science in shaping the presumptions that are brought to bear on cultural interpretation. Schneider critiques the over-reliance on such presumptions, whereas Weiner points out the obfuscations they impose not only in the understanding of other cultures' reproductive models, but of our own. Both of these perspectives anticipate later, more explicit, attention to the role of biology as a cultural system.

In her cogent reassessment of the 'virgin birth' debates from the point of view of why it was so important to anthropologists to begin with, Carol Delaney offered an important set of refractions on this fractious legacy in the mid-1980s. Following Weiner, Delaney argued that biological reproduction *simply wasn't the point* for the Australians or the Trobrianders. That it *was the only point* for anthropologists simply constitutes a very clear case of mis-conception. This slippage is overdetermined. Paternity, Delaney argued, is not 'primarily physiological'. It is not 'automatically a natural fact'. Instead, 'paternity is a concept, the meaning of which is derived from its interrelations with other concepts and beliefs'. Rather than being 'a categorical entity, the presence or absence of which can be determined empirically', it is a 'conceptual relation' (Delaney 1986: 495).

Delaney suggested that the model of paternity ascribed to by anthropologists derives from the Judaeo-Christian 'cultural logic' of monogenetic, or single-source, creation. As Christian divinity is modelled on one God who created all life, so too does paternity do conceptual service in Judaeo-Christian and other monotheistic societies for the power to create in general. Paternity, she suggests, is not the semantic equivalent of maternity: in the Judaeo-Christian tradition, paternity has meant begetting, and maternity has meant bearing. The dominant idiom for this difference is of 'the seed and the soil': 'the child originates with the father, from his seed' (1986: 497). The over-reliance on this concept of paternity, she argues, is exemplified in the 'virgin birth' debate. In Delaney's view, Leach completely overlooked the significance of the fact that paternity has been used to describe 'the male generative role in the production of a child . . . as *the* generative and creative one' (1986: 501). The whole point of Leach's comparison between the Virgin Birth and the procreative beliefs of the Trobrianders was their mutual denial of physical paternity. But this is not a valid point of comparison if the Trobrianders have no conceptual equivalent to paternity, as begetting, at all.

Likewise, Malinowski did not follow his own advice to avoid glossing the Trobriand kinship term *tama* as 'father'. This led only to confusions, as he predicted it would. Instead of exploring how 'fatherhood' or 'paternity' would appear through *tama* identities, Delaney argues, 'he concentrated on finding a place for the male' (1986: 505) and on reconciling the Trobriand models to those of 'physical paternity'. In contrast, she points out, Weiner emphasises that the *dala*, or matriline, is described as a continuous embodiment of identity that is not so much *created* as *recreated* and maintained. Echoing Malinowski, Delaney concludes that 'because of [their] lack of attention . . . anthropologists lost an important opportunity to see that procreative beliefs in Western culture are as much a cultural construction as those of the Trobrianders' (1986: 508).

Delaney's suggestion that 'it is the anthropologists who have not understood the meaning of paternity' (1986: 494) invited a deeper reconsideration of the role of the cultural givens which have structured anthropological inquiry in the area of conception theory. This invitation closely paralleled Yanagisako's argument that it is the 'biological facts of reproduction' which have been 'at the core of our studies of the cultural organization of gender, at the same time that [they constitute] the core of the genealogical grid that has defined kinship' (1985: 1). The first set of consequences of this argument works at the level of visibility, in the form of a challenge to the relegation of certain questions to the realm of the 'mere biological'. What has been most taken for granted, Yanagisako argued, is what most needs to be explained.

Arguing in their co-edited 1995 volume, *Naturalizing Power*, Yanagisako and Delaney propose that:

> In Darwinian theory the natural order retained both the hierarchical order of [Biblical] Creation and its god-given quality; the difference is that the power no longer came from God, it came from Nature. . . . The secularization of the hierarchical order of Creation was exemplified in social evolutionary models such as that constructed by Morgan. . . . Kinship, which has been at the core of anthropology since the nineteenth century, has been a primary site for the development of a natural progression that echoes the hierarchical order inherent in the Great Chain of Being.
> (Yanagisako and Delaney 1995: 5–6)

This has essential consequences for Euro-American understandings of sexuality, reproduction and gender, they argue, which 'are held to be quintessentially natural activities' (1995: 6). It is the ubiquitous naturalisation of reproduction which has rendered it inaccessible to certain kinds of investigation, they suggest. It also has specific consequences for gender: once reproduction 'has been reduced to its natural character and is associated with women; women have been defined by and confined to their reproductive role' (1995: 9). The male role in reproduction, on the other hand, has been 'abstracted and generalized as creativity, productivity, genius' (1995: 9).[20]

A related consequence of 'naturalisation' operates through what Strathern has described as 'domaining', whereby borders are drawn between distinctive domains of thought or belief, maintaining their separation, as in the distinction between religion and science. A similar practice, Yanagisako and Delaney argue, has characterised the traditional ('objectified') view of culture as 'something that exists apart from representational politics of those who employ this concept' (1995: 15). Following Abu-Lughod, they suggest an ethnographic representational politics of 'writing against culture', by challenging the notion of discrete domains, such as science. In contrast, Yanagisako and Delaney advocate a model of 'reading across cultural domains that are defined as separate . . . especially those which are supposedly independent of social life and whose truths are said to be rooted in nature' (1995: 14).

The implications of both Yanagisako's and Delaney's arguments in the mid-1980s concerning the operation of biological models is thus spelled out in the mid-1990s as a major project of *denaturalisation*. Their main aim in assembling the contents of *Naturalizing Power* is to draw attention to the 'ways in which differentials of power come already embedded in culture' through which 'power appears natural, inevitable, even god-given' (1995: 1). This project is thus one of *defamiliarisation*, whereby familiar legitimations of both specific phenomena, such as reproduction, and the analytical domaining of such phenomena, for example as 'natural' or 'biological', can be challenged.

This project thus responds to the problem of the 'hidden' operations of naturalisation, for which the 'virgin birth' debates are a prime example. However, this broad objective has many components. An important question signalled by both Yanagisako and Delaney's introduction, and the contents of their anthology, is the need to specify in more substantial detail what kinds of representational 'work' naturalisations achieve, and how their social negotiation corresponds, or does not correspond, to their operations as 'hegemonic' cultural systems. This involves moving beyond the project undertaken by Emily Martin in the mid-1980s to examine the dominant scientific construction of reproduction, and the question of whether women understand themselves in relation to such models (1987). In particular, this project requires attention to the processes by which dominant scientific models of, for example, the 'biological facts' of reproduction are constituted in and through more popular cultural forms, as Martin demonstrates in her witty and trenchant account of 'The Egg and the Sperm' (1991).

One set of consequences of the need to denaturalise reproduction thus invokes a social field. As Rayna Rapp described it: 'Once we culturalize, rather than naturalize, women, the social space in which "biological" experiences are constructed is intimately shared with other social relations' (1982: 7). In her work on the social negotiation of prenatal screening, Rapp has extended this insight to provide one of the most substantial ethnographic portraits of 'biology' as a cultural system ever undertaken by an anthropologist (forthcoming). Like Ginsburg's pioneering work on contestations over abortion (1989), such ethnographic documentation has been essential to the removal of reproduction from its former invisibility as a site of potent cultural meanings. In turn, this effort has resulted in a recent resurgence of interest in the anthropology of reproduction, a project to which this volume is also contributing (see Davis-Floyd and Sargent 1996; Franklin and Ragone 1997; Ginsburg and Rapp 1995).

Yet another set of consequences of the project to 'denaturalise' reproduction concerns the operations of biology as a cultural system, or as a discourse. It is on this point that Yanagisako argued Schneider 'did not go far enough'. An approach to this problem is through the history of biology as a science, as was initially explored by Barnes (1973). Like Delaney, Barnes argued that:

> The main stream of Western popular belief has clearly been "one child, one genitor" .... Likewise the Christian faith of the West stresses the uniqueness of God the Father .... If we encountered this constellation of facts in a tribal society, surely we would have no hesitation in saying that the organization of society and the major premises of religion are reflected in myths about unique physical parenthood.
>
> (Barnes 1973: 68)

Unlike Delaney, however, Barnes reached this conclusion on the basis of how little has been known about physical paternity within the history of western science. He points out, for example, that not only is there a wide range of orthodox scientific theories supporting poly-paternity in the past, but that 'there is evidence double fertilization sometimes occurs naturally in humans' (1973: 67). He adds that:

> The process of marsupial gestation remained a mystery long after the White settlement [of Australia] in 1788. Although the unaided passage of a kangaroo embryo from the vagina towards the pouch was recorded in 1830, more than a hundred years later many Australians firmly believed that marsupial young develop on teats "like apples on twigs". . . . There is no reason why Aboriginals should have based their ethnoscience of human reproduction on the euthrial dingo or bat any more than the kangaroo or other ubiquitous marsupials.
>
> (Barnes 1973: 71, see also Sharman and Pilton 1964)

Much as this analysis reaches for evidence to support the view that biology is a cultural system, it is, as the title suggests ('Genitrix: Genitor: : Nature: Culture'), very similar to Ortner's argument, with which this chapter began. All of the evident uncertainty available from both the 'folk models' and orthodox scientific views of paternity which might lead Barnes to conclude differently are revealed at the penultimate moment to support his view that: 'the mother–child relation in nature is plain to see and necessary for individual survival . . . [and] is at least in some degree innate or genetically-determined' (1973: 73). Hence, he is arguing in time-honoured fashion, that *mater semper certa est* and that 'some aspects of nature impinge more obviously and insistently on the human imagination than others' (1973: 73).

The investigation of the history of biology as a cultural system thus falls, at present, largely outside anthropology. That even the Darwinian model of genealogy is drawn from the Judaeo-Christian image of the 'tree of life', however, suggests the importance of studies which combine attention to the history of European folk, religious and scientific models of nature, life, conception, procreation and kinship with the history of anthropology. In her detailed historical work on the concordances between the early iconography of the Tree of Jesse, its similarity to the tree iconography introduced by Haeckel in the 1860s to represent evolutionary linkages, and the genealogical method introduced by Rivers, Mary Bouquet provides a stunning example of how deeply embedded are the 'tools of the anthropological trade' in the history of European culture. She writes:

> Anthropology *out* of the original contexts in which it was studied provides fresh insight – another perspective – on the ethnographic assumptions of those original locations and, indeed, on the very tools of the trade (such as the genealogical method) forged there.
>
> (Bouquet 1994: 14)

Retracing the family trees, the genealogies and pedigrees of anthropological knowledge responds to both intellectual and political necessities in the 'retooling' of late-twentieth century anthropology. In particular, the cultural dimensions of European science provide an important perspective on the origins of origin models and their accompanying artefacts.

By making explicit the inadequacy of the 'biological facts of human reproduction' as the given ground for both kinship and gender theory, Yanagisako brought about what Marilyn Strathern has described as an effect of 'literalisation'. This is 'a mode of laying out the coordinates or conventional points of reference of what is otherwise taken for granted' (Strathern 1992a: 5). The effects of making explicit, or literalisation, are several. One effect is of displacement: once the taken-for-granteds are made explicit, they no longer function as they did. The second effect is of substitution: new ideas take the place of the ones displaced by literalisation. In attempting to describe a sense of epoch, Strathern argues it is just these sorts of practices which create the sense of being post-, or after the fact, definitive of the present.

Like Strathern's approach, which seeks to 'use British anthropological kinship theory and English kin constructs as mutual perspectives on each other's modernisms' (1992a: 8), this book attempts to examine an effect of displacement. The 'biological facts' of reproduction have not only been displaced from their former status as given within anthropology, they have become more publicly contingent and uncertain as a part of social life. Complementing Strathern, who argues this has had a 'flattening' effect on the nature-culture opposition which structured so many Euro-American taken-for-granteds – including those of British kinship theory, Paul Rabinow has suggested a similar process. Culture, he argues, now serves as the model for nature, which is, through the life sciences, now 'known and remade as technique and will finally become artificial, just as culture becomes natural' (1992: 242).

Like the work of both Strathern and Bouquet, this book situates its argument in relation to the refractory turn provided by anthropology's own origins in examining its accounts of 'coming into being'. Developing upon the insights of Yanagisako and Delaney, it explores the ways in which 'narratives of origin tell people what kind of world it is, what it consists of, and where they stand in it' (1994: 1). Like Haraway's powerful accounts of Euro-American origin stories in both primatology and embryology (1976, 1989), this book situates contemporary accounts of conception within the history of their anthropological explanation, inviting new forms of 'traffic' between the two domains.

In the following chapters, I explore the elucidation of such questions by attending to the social negotiation of such shifts. In addition to studying the effects of literalisation and displacement, this study also attempts to examine some of the processses of substitution consequent upon a loss of certainty about 'the facts of life'. What are the responses of clinicians, infertile couples, parliamentarians and journalists to this loss? What are the explanations, analogies and imagery introduced to substitute for what has been displaced? How can such changes be investigated through the analysis of emergent cultural forms? Although this study is not intended to be read as an 'ethnography', and lacks many of the conventional characteristics of that genre, it retains a commitment to the value of empirically grounded cultural analysis, and it engages directly with questions of anthropological representation. It thus contributes to the ethnographic perspectives offered by Rapp, Ginsburg and Ragone in asking not only how forms of displacement or literalisation affect our ability to conceive of culture, but what form of methodological perspective this might entail. How might ethnographic representation work in relation to the production of cultural theory, when the ethnographic subjects share the same confusions as the anthropologists? Of what significance is the ongoing redefinition of families and their relatives in England to the project of their reinvention within Euro-American anthropology? Keeping the 'virgin birth' debates in the background, with their conceptual apparatus now literalised as a relational perspective on their own origins, Chapter 2 introduces less familiar uncertainties about 'the facts of life' and their contested meanings.

Chapter 2

Contested conceptions in the enterprise culture

INTRODUCTION

The scale of cultural difference for an American in England can at first be apprehended in terms of sheer size. The effect is of miniaturisation. Familiar objects, such as grocery carts or automobiles, appear bizarrely small. They are reduced to a proportion of their former self. It was quite fascinating to encounter, for example, refrigerators that were in every respect identical to those found in American homes, only much tinier. Inside these tiny refrigerators were even tinier freezer compartments. And the tiniest ice cube trays I had ever seen inhabited those tiny freezers. The ice cubes were the size of dice. This impression of 'matchbox' England was particularly pronounced when airborne: the neatness of the rows of houses, and their uniformity, contributing to an odd sense of familiarity offset by shifts of perspective. Such shifts became familiar to me in England, which is, as they say, divided from America by a common language.

Returning to the United States produced the reverse effect. I was astounded by the enormity of cereal boxes. I was out of the habit of consumer choice, and overwhelmed by the orange juice selections. Ordering a cup of coffee reminded me how much consumer knowledge is required for everyday transactions in America: caffeinated or decaffeinated? small, medium or large? milk or cream? sugar or sweet 'n low? to stay or to go? with a lid or without a lid? Do you want it in a bag? Things were simpler in England – the coffee wasn't worth ordering, if it was available at all. I could buy more varieties of crumpets in Boston than I had ever seen in Brighton or Birmingham. I was becoming mid-Atlantic.

In his characteristically elegant and wise reflections on *The Country and the City*, Raymond Williams describes how the contrast between them reproduces itself over time, creating the effect of being on a moving escalator, aboard which 'Old England', so recently left behind ('Just back, we can see, over the last hill') keeps pace, like a never-receding horizon. The point of reference which remains fixed is not the land itself but the 'structures of feeling' towards it which create a nostalgia for the past that is lost, like the old cobbles beneath the tarmac. He notes, 'the initial problem is one of perspective' (1973: 9). The contrast between America and Britain also works as a never-receding horizon; like the ocean between them, it is always flowing back and forth. Like the country and the city, this contrast is so established as to itself have become a kind of semiotic engine, always being used to generate one point of view or another, to ground some claim about similarity or difference, better or worse, older or newer, right or wrong. This is another way to find the mid-Atlantic.

As Strathern has noted, 'the stable and the transient coexist in a manner that makes it possible to ask, of almost anything, how much change has taken place. This is a very general, ordinary and otherwise unremarkable kind of question. It seems to lead naturally to further questions about what should be conserved and what should be reformed' (1992a: 2). Like Williams's comparison of the country and the city, Strathern notes how much continuity and change depend upon one another to make visible either effect. She too would describe this as a question of perspective. The 'Americanisation' of Britain under Thatcher, so often referred to on both sides of the Atlantic in the 1980s, is a comparison of this sort. It establishes a perspective that is only ever grounded in the never-receding horizon of a cultural difference which eludes the very fixity it seeks to affirm. As Strathern describes it: 'the mechanisms might be simple, but the products or results were innumerable' (1992a: 8). I offer this brief qualification of the following account of cultural change in 1980s Britain simply out of caution, for it too comprises the imposition of a perspective that might, from another shore, be as easily unmoored.

THATCHERISM AND THE ENTERPRISE CULTURE OF 1980s BRITAIN

Margaret Thatcher was elected in 1979 and won two re-elections to remain the leader of the British government for eleven years, abruptly being deposed by her party in 1990.[1] During the 1980s she brought about far reaching changes in British society, prevailing as one of the most successful and powerful politicians of her era. 'Thatcherism' was a term that became established to describe the singularity of the social transformations underway in Britain in the 1980s and their identification with the singular character of the Prime Minister herself. These changes included a wholesale redefinition of citizenship, national identity and the social contract between the Government and the nation's population.[2] Like Reagan, with whom she was closely allied ideologically, 'Mrs T', as she was popularly known, sought to combine neo-liberal economic policies emphasising maximum market freedom, and conservative moral values, particularly in relation to the family. Thatcher was even more successful than Reagan in bringing about these changes because the British welfare state left more room for change in the direction both she and Reagan favoured, and in part because she was in power longer and her party had control of Parliament while she was in office. The American equivalent would have been an eleven year reign by Ronald Reagan with the Republicans holding a clear Congressional majority throughout and presiding over about one-quarter of the US population.[3]

During her Prime Ministership, Thatcher enjoyed enormous popularity and was particularly widely revered among large sections of the working class population. Much to the chagrin of her opponents in the Labour Party, Thatcher seized and held the support of a large section of Labour's traditional constituency. In part, this was because the form of conservatism Thatcher advocated was less 'Shire Tory', or conservative-aristocratic, and more 'authoritarian populist', to use Stuart Hall's description (1988). Thatcher's conservatism was radical: her cornershop, lower-middle class upbringing served as her baseline political point of reference throughout her career, and it was modelled on self-reliance. In the service of a vision of an 'enterprise culture' which became a hallmark of Thatcherism, the 'Iron Lady' was utterly dedicated to transforming British national identity down to the level of its basic commonsense components. She went about this task with a fierce determination that held enormous charismatic appeal and hugely enhanced her popularity as a single-minded, unequivocal and defiant leader.

The main targets of Thatcherite political transformation were the institutions and the 'culture' of the welfare state. Under Thatcher, the British national industries including coal, electricity and gas were privatised, and the branches of the welfare state, including health, education and social services, were significantly reduced. What was left of them was restructured to function on a more entrepreneurial basis, through Draconian management procedures designed to maximise efficiency of provision and to minimise cost to the taxpayer. Alongside this reduction of services went the Thatcherite 'war of position' against the so-called 'dependency culture' fostered by years of purported over-reliance on government subsidies. Demonising every vestigial remnant of 'state-sponsored socialism', Thatcher simply abolished as much as she legally could, and cut down the rest to the greatest degree possible.

In so doing, Thatcher met her greatest resistance in relation to the National Health Service (NHS), for which the British public held a deep appreciation including a sense of national pride. The NHS remained under Thatcher one of the most efficient in the world, comprising less than 6 per cent of GNP in 1988, or 14.7 per cent of public expenditure (Pearson 1992: 218). None the less, rising healthcare costs internationally, produced by a larger population of elderly patients, and rising expenditure related to new high-technology medical treatments, mean that governments of many nations are seeking to control this sector more stringently. Thatcher imposed restrictions on the NHS aimed to enforce maximum cost reduction, and she simultaneously encouraged the growth of the private healthcare sector. The privatisation of health was encouraged both within the NHS, by making it easier for GPs to take private patients while retaining their full NHS salaries, and outside the NHS by encouraging the growth of private healthcare schemes. Until Thatcherism, the private healthcare market in Britain was extremely small, with three companies controlling 98 per cent of market share. From 4.2 per cent of the population, or just over one million private healthcare subscribers in 1975, the figures had more than doubled by 1988 to 8.8 per cent, or 2.3 million subscribers (Pearson 1992: 221).

The rapid expansion of private healthcare, combined with the increasing amount of private practice among NHS GPs and specialists raised vociferous public outcry, and became one of the most fractious issues for the Thatcher government. The widely perceived decline in the quality of service provided by the NHS, which was consistently challenged by government statistics, came to symbolise the failures of Thatcherism across a wide segment of the population. In particular, the increasing number of patients who could afford to 'queue jump' by arranging private appointments with their GP, or who could afford to opt out of NHS care altogether by joining private-healthcare schemes, led to accusations of a return to the 'two-tiered' health system that existed before the NHS was formed in 1943. This in turn came to symbolise the iniquities fostered under the Thatcherite 'culture of enterprise' which was seen to undermine both the moral fabric of the nation and the basic right to healthcare of its population, especially those of limited means.

Offsetting the public discontent raised by cuts to the NHS, and also to education, was the enormous popularity of Thatcherite reform of the housing sector. Seeking both to reduce public expenditure on housing, and to increase the number of home-owners in Britain, the Thatcher government passed the Right to Buy Act in 1980, enabling tenants living in homes owned by local councils to purchase them at discount rates. This option, combined with attractive mortgage rates and tax-relief on mortgage payments, was among several factors contributing to a property boom in Britain during the 1980s. The net result was a substantial increase in both property values and home ownership. The percentage of owner-occupied housing rose from 54 per cent in 1979 to 67 per cent in 1990, accompanied by a rise in the UK average house price from £20,000 to £67,000 in the same period. Mortgage debt also increased, from £45 to £275 billion, corresponding with a rise in both foreclosure and homelessness (Williams 1992: 166–7). However, the downside of the Thatcherite reform of housing was not nearly as visible or contentious among the general public as was her reform of the NHS. Instead, house purchase came to symbolise for important sectors of the Thatcherite constituency exactly the benefits of the enterprise culture she aimed to illustrate, namely greater consumer choice as a result of greater market freedom, benefitting 'individuals and their families'.

The Thatcherite aim of creating a 'nation of home-owners' and a 'share-owning democracy' distilled her primary ideological goal of redefining citizenship along the analogy of customers seeking services. Against the 'dependency culture' of the welfare state she aimed to encourage 'self-reliance' through precisely such activities as home purchase and purchase of shares in the former national industries she privatised. In what has become one of her most famous phrases, Thatcher claimed there was 'no such thing as society, there are only individuals and their families'. The model of the working-class family 'buying out' of their dependency on local council housing, and 'buying in' to the Thatcherite consumer-analogy for citizenship precisely expressed her ideal relation of government to the governed, which was minimal. It also expressed her view that just as markets work best, and therefore most fairly, when they are unhampered by government regulation, so people work best when they are striving on behalf of their own individual and their family's benefit.

The increase in home ownership, accompanied by the steep rise in house prices generated by the market expansion this 'jump start' catalysed, realised enormous financial gains for a limited, but still large, sector of the population, many of whom had never imagined they would benefit from this source of capital accumulation. Although the tarnished legacy of this housing boom has become apparent in the form of widespread negative equity in the 1990s, the rosier side of the housing market held sway throughout the 1980s. In contrast to the NHS, housing proved a very successful chapter for Thatcherism and literally brought home many of its core tenets.

ASSISTED CONCEPTION IN THE ENTERPRISE CULTURE

These two features of the Thatcherite redefinition of British citizenship during the 1980s had important consequences for the population discussed in this study, who were consumers of private healthcare, aiming to produce a family, on whose behalf they could exercise the kinds of consumer choices valorised within the enterprise culture. For Thatcher, the right to exercise choice in general, and consumer choice in particular, was the carrot at the end of the anti-welfare state stick. Reproductive choice fits neatly into this equation. Consumers of private reproductive medicine in Britain during the 1980s were able both to take advantage of the many clinics eager to establish themselves in this rapidly expanding sector, and, indirectly of the tax incentives provided by the government to encourage such entrepreneurial activity. Although assisted conception was not 'big business' in Britain in the immediate wake of the birth of Louise Brown in 1978, by the mid-1980s it had gained momentum, and by the late 1980s it was expanding very rapidly.[4] In the city of Birmingham alone, the number of IVF clinics tripled from two to six between 1986 and 1989. The 'enterprising up' of conception thus exemplified the broader context of celebratory political initiatives aimed to enhance entrepreneurial activity, and consequently widen consumer choice.

Although some IVF clinics were established within large, urban NHS hospitals in cities such as London, Manchester and Birmingham, these were an exception to the rule of largely private services on offer.[5] At a time of cuts to the NHS, infertility services were not a priority, and without the efforts of individual consultants who prioritised this area, they were unlikely to be offered through NHS hospitals. In the private sector, on the other hand, IVF could be offered at especially low rates due to the possibility of having the necessary prescriptions for expensive hormone dosages met through a woman's own NHS GP. Since these expensive pharmaceutical products account for nearly half the overall cost of each IVF cycle, clients of private reproductive healthcare in Britain essentially received a large government subsidy for treatment.[6] This made IVF more affordable in Britain than it is, for example, in the US. Still, the average cost of a cycle at several hundred pounds made it available to a limited population.

During preparation for this study, I conducted observations in both a large NHS fertility clinic, and a private clinical facility nearby. The contrast between these two facilities underscored the accusations of a 'two-tiered' system raised by many critics during Thatcher's leadership. NHS hospitals in Britain offer excellent healthcare, comparable to that of any other wealthy industrialised nation. The high quality of this provision, however, is not reflected in the quality of service through which it is dispatched. The relation might more accurately be described as inversely proportionate. The service ethos is not deeply instilled in Britain in general, and, under extraordinary pressures to increase their levels of provision, NHS hospitals were not a good place to look for a 'warm and cuddly feeling' approach to customer provision.

Although this situation has changed in Britain in the context of expansive growth in the service sector, the 'how can I be of service' mentality (which has far fewer derogatory connotations in the US than in the UK) has hardly become second nature to most British service-sector employees. This was especially evident in large NHS hospitals, where the provision of 'care' did not include customer service niceties. Institutionally, these large hospitals had a worn, threadbare look about them, and the waiting rooms looked more like they belonged in an Aeroflot terminal than a worldclass medical facility. Hard, plastic chairs of indeterminate vintage, style or colour typically lined the walls beneath bulletin boards covered with public health advice and posters. Since fertility services within the NHS are often run as part of wider Ob-Gyn clinics, the rooms where women undergoing IVF waited to be seen were mostly filled with pregnant women. Most of the waiting time was for hormone injections or ultrasound monitoring. For these procedures there was minimal privacy, and the nurses were brisk and brusque at best. Long delays were common, as were long faces, and the general feeling was not very cheerful. The descriptions many women gave of NHS clinics as 'cattle markets' are perhaps extreme, but they were not unwarranted.

The NHS nurses with whom I spent most of my time were working under quite extreme conditions, and for very low pay. Like teachers, nurses remain among the lowest paid of trained professionals in public service in Britain. Whereas the clinic staff in private IVF programmes tended to see themselves more as a 'team', with a specialised professional function, which included making an effort to leave customers feeling looked after, the NHS clinics were far more hierarchical, overstretched, under-resourced and highly pressured. The NHS nurses' sense of humour was correspondingly irreverent and hard-hitting. In their private station, just out of sight of the room full of waiting patients, they told outrageous anecdotes and wickedly teased the (all male) doctors. Although I always enjoyed my time at the NHS hospital far more than at the private clinics, it was certainly not a place I would have wanted to visit as a patient, or to work as a health professional.

The private clinic I observed in and those I visited were quite the opposite in terms of physical facilities, 'customer services' and the attitudes of staff towards their patients/clients. In private hospitals, the floors were carpeted, the woman behind the information desk was courteous and helpful, and the general impression was more like domestic than institutional space. The hallways were neat, quiet and well-lit, with not a trace of the dull, scratched linoleum characteristic of NHS hospitals. If anything overdecorated, much like middle-class domestic English sitting rooms, the feel of private clinics was typically of newly-furnished, up-market, plush-but-not-posh surroundings. These clinics had an eager-to-please atmosphere, consistent with their eagerness to increase market share.

SETTING UP THE STUDY

The clinic through which participants for the study were contacted was in a private medical facility in a wealthy suburb on the outskirts of a large city in England. It was one of several IVF clinics in the area, all of which were recently opened. Of the twenty-two women and couples interviewed for this study, all were middle class in terms of their present standard of living, if not by upbringing. All were white, married and in their mid-thirties to mid-forties. The homo-geneity of this group in part reflects the conditions of access to IVF, in particular its cost. Although marriage is not a requirement for access to IVF, the medical director of the clinic had strong views about the naturalness of the reproductive drive, and it is likely unmarried or non-heterosexual women would not have felt welcome, if they were allowed onto the programme at all. Legally, the question of assisted conception provision for single or lesbian women was being debated in Parliament at the time of the study (1989–90). It was therefore of unclear legitimacy which undoubtedly exercised a 'chilling effect' in relation to potentially 'unacceptable' clients.[7]

Ethnically, the interview pool was not representative of the wider population of IVF consumers, as there is a significant Black and Asian clientele in Britain who use assisted conception services.[8] At some clinics, such as the premiere private British facility at Bourne Hall, founded by Robert Edwards and Patrick Steptoe, a large and diverse international clientele is served. IVF is itself very well established internationally, having as long a history in India, for example, as in Britain, Australia or the United States. It is by no means a 'western' practice, although it is everywhere a technique largely restricted to those who can pay for it, and thus highly differentiated by class.

Systematic data on the women interviewed in terms of personal characteristics such as religious preference, educational level, house-hold income, or family history were not collected for this study, in which identifying characteristics were kept to a minimum for reasons of privacy. Since this was not a quantitative study, such data were not considered necessary. Moreover, considerable concern was expressed by participants that their identities should be protected, and even the original letter sent out by the clinic requesting participa-tion in the study caused a degree of discomfort among many of the clients not interviewed, and some who were. Although more detailed correlations between, for example, religious preferences and inter-pretations of assisted conception, would no doubt have been reveal-ing, such questions could also evoke defensive responses, or refusals to answer, and I have focused very closely on the technique of IVF itself in this study.

I explained to the interviewees that I was conducting a study on in vitro fertilisation with a view to understanding better the specific-ally social and cultural (rather than medical) dimensions of the technique. I suggested this data might at some point comprise a basis for comparative studies, for example in relation to infertility treatment in the US, and that in any event the study aimed to identify key issues for women and couples undergoing IVF. When asked specifically about my methodology, I sometimes described this study as a 'factor-finding search,' hoping to indicate I was not entirely sure what I was looking for and relied on them to tell me. Most often, they were more interested in why a young American woman would move to Britain.

The option to be interviewed alone or with their spouse was left open, and only a quarter of the interviews were with couples.[9] Most of the women interviewed had significant experience of paid work outside the home, and many had active professional careers as teachers, nurses, social workers and secretaries. Eighty-five per cent of respondents claimed that paid work outside the home had helped them cope with the demands of infertility treatment. However, a majority of 75 per cent had either already left, or were planning to leave, full-time employment as a result of the choice to opt for IVF. The women interviewed also worked, or had recently worked, as childminders, assembly-line workers, managers and saleswomen, and thus as a group represented a wide range of work experience. The average number of years spent in previous infertility treatment was five, with a total of over a century of treatment amongst the group as a whole. The average number of years women had been married at the time of the interviews was nine.

Not all of the women interviewed were childless. Two had biological children and one had a GIFT baby by donation. Neither were all of the women infertile, with three undergoing treatment because of their partner's infertility. In the remaining cases, reasons for treatment varied: in seven cases resulting from blocked tubes; eight from unexplained infertility; and four with multiple factors that were shared. The average number of IVF cycles already undertaken by the time of the interview was three, with ten being the highest and one woman having become pregnant on her first attempt. Five of the women interviewed were pregnant at the time of the interview, producing a 25 per cent pregnancy rate overall. This was much higher than the average UK success rate at the time of this study, which was 8.6 per cent (Voluntary Licensing Authority 1988). This figure may reflect a greater tendency for women who had been successful to agree to an interview, although not all of the women pregnant at the time of the interview knew so at the time of their initial consent to participate in the study. It has also to be assumed that not all of the women who became pregnant would necessarily give birth, and there was no follow-up to this study to determine overall live birth rates.[10]

A very high percentage, 95 per cent, of the women interviewed were well aware of the low success rate of IVF before they decided to attempt it. Few, however, knew very much about the potential side-effects or health hazards of the drugs used in this technique.[11] When asked about side-effects, only four women mentioned any at all, all of which were discounted as minimal. Similarly, when asked about the risk of multiple births, although well aware of this possibility, no concerns were expressed by the respondents, who if anything viewed such a prospect as a bonus.[12] In terms of alternatives to IVF, only one respondent had not considered adoption: the remaining 95 per cent had given it considerable thought, but had either experienced or been warned of difficulties, in particular their age and the limited supply of children available for adoption in their particular region. A significant majority, of 95 per cent, praised the clinic where they were undergoing treatment and expressed a high level of consumer satisfaction. Both the medical and the support staff were lavishly praised and comparisons to unpleasant experiences of fertility treatment on the NHS were frequently invoked in support of the clinic.

As a group, therefore, the women interviewed could be described as well-informed, generally highly educated and/or professionally trained, in long-term conjugal relationships, and very positive about their choice to opt for IVF, and the clinic where they were attempting it. They were on the whole articulate, well-informed, reflective about their experiences and highly self-aware. I never encountered any difficulties discussing a sensitive, painful and often quite intimate topic with any of the women or couples, as they were enormously forthright, generous and self-assured in the context of being interviewed. Likewise, they exercised a great deal of control over the interview – refusing to answer questions, and asking me to clarify myself, when necessary. Although I always enjoyed the interviews, they were exhausting.

My aim was to interview women in the midst of treatment, and they were initially contacted through the clinic by mail. A letter explaining the study and an enclosed reply sheet were enclosed in the mailing, which was sent to eighty-five women. Twenty-five replied affirmatively, of which twenty-two were interviewed with five of the husbands in the 1988–9 academic year. For the interview, they were given a choice of meeting at the clinic or in their homes, although none chose to be interviewed at the clinic. The home-interview visits were arranged by phone, at which time I took directions to their houses, some of which were over an hour's drive from the clinic. Navigating these routes, often at night, in my co-owned, ancient, manual transmission, Austin Allegro, I marvelled often at the dedication it required to travel such routes daily in the course of treatment.

I was always relieved to find their homes and to have avoided once again the engine failure I was certain would beset me at some point in my labyrinthian nocturnal motorings. Happily, no such mechanical failures compromised my interview schedule, which proceeded apace over the better part of a year. Once arrived, I was always met with a warmth, hospitality and openness that very much impressed me. Tea was always offered and the interviews always took place in the sitting room. I explained the interview in roughly chronological fashion. I was interested in how they first became aware of their infertility, how they decided to choose IVF, what their experience of treatment had been like, and how things were going just at the moment. I explained I was researching for a book about IVF, and that what I was mostly interested in was their own personal experiences of treatment.[13] I asked permission to tape record the interviews, and I had a short list of prompts I would use to make sure I covered certain details, for example who they told about their infertility and/or treatment, how they found out about the clinic, and what their advice to other women who might want to undergo the procedure would be. Usually, I hardly needed to say very much at all once the interviews began, since they were set up to elicit openended accounts and my main role was simply to listen. Often the experience of retelling their personal stories brought women to tears, for this was on the whole a painful and difficult subject to discuss. I gained enormous respect for the courage and determination of the women and men I interviewed, and I continue to feel an indebtedness to their openness, honesty and generosity I hope this book will go at least some way towards repaying.

Because of the intensity of the subject matter, the length of the interviews, and the nervewracking process of getting to and from my destinations, I was inevitably exhausted after each encounter. A different, calmer, though equally intense mental exertion is generated by the transcription process, which involves a literal retracing of every utterance. The results of these interviews, presented in the next three chapters, provide a detailed portrait of IVF. Although I do not claim this account as representative, for the sample size was very small, I do suggest it is indicative of many core elements of IVF as 'a way of life'. In particular, the extent to which the technique 'takes over' a woman's life is clearly evident in these accounts, which, though I seek carefully to situate them in a particular time and place, are in fact similar to those encountered by other researchers.[14]

Additional studies would greatly enhance the comparative dimension to the cultural understanding of assisted conception. Specifically, studies involving a more ethnically diverse population would be of great value, as would studies of women and couples who chose not to undergo assisted conception. A follow-up study to this account would also have been of enormous value, in assessing the changing evaluations of treatment over time. Greater attention to the trade-off between the choice to opt for IVF and for adoption would also repay further investigation. Although the present study was in all of these respects limited, as such intensive studies always are, certain of the findings presented here are distinctive. In particular, the consistent finding in every interview of women's sense that they 'had to choose' IVF was so striking as to merit careful foregrounding in the analysis I offer in the following chapters. This proved a central and important finding, which, though confined by other studies (especially Sandelowski), is given particular attention here.

THE BROADER CONTEXT OF PUBLIC DEBATE

The timing of this study coincided not only with the peak of 'Thatcherism', but also with the culmination of an intensive public debate of human fertilisation and embryology in Britain, which had begun with the birth of Louise Brown in 1978. Though Louise Brown was less than a year old when Thatcher came to power, she would be nearly a teenager before the British government established legislation governing the use of assisted conception technologies. I have elsewhere discussed in depth the parliamentary debate of the Human Fertilisation and Embryology Act (Franklin 1993a), and will not belabour its lengthy and prolix evolution here. However, a few rudimentary details are useful.[15]

With the birth of Louise Brown via unprecedented scientific methods was also seen to be born 'a legal vacuum' that needed to be filled. The first effort to redress this absence was the formation of the Warnock Committee in 1982, set up to advise the government, Parliament and the general public on the matter of human fertil- isation and embryology. This phrasing is significant, as it fore- grounds a single event, 'human fertilisation', and an area of scientific knowledge describing a developmental process, 'embryology'. What was significant to these debates, as in so much of the history of social theory which has preceded them, were the specific details of the conceptive process, and their consequences for social and political organisation. This precise phrasing remained consistent, as the title of the 1990 'Human Fertilisation and Embryology Act' makes clear. Headed by the philosopher Mary Warnock, the so-called *Warnock Report* was published in 1984. It made various recommendations including the establishment of a licensing body to oversee develop- ments and provision in the area of reproductive medicine, the establishment of criteria governing the status of children born of new techniques, and the criteria for legal limits on research on human fertilisation and embryology. In 1986, the government produced a Consultation Paper aimed to elicit input from the general public and various concerned parties and organisations (DHSS 1986). In 1987, a White Paper was published outlining proposed legislation (DHSS 1987). This did not go before Parliament until 1989, when it was debated, amended and, in the autumn of 1990, enacted.

In the course of its debate in Parliament, two especially contentious issues arose. Although the general public overwhelmingly supported the use of IVF and the implantation of 'test-tube' embryos (by 83 per cent in 1985 and by 85 per cent in 1987, Harding 1988: 39), they were much more sceptical towards any technique involving an 'outside' party. Commercial surrogacy was the most highly pub- licised incidence of 'third party' reproduction, and was banned in 1985 under the Surrogacy Arrangements Act. In response to a private American surrogacy-arrangement agency attempting to set up busi- ness in London (Noel Keane), the 'enterprise culture' went into reverse gear, calling on traditional family values and the limits of commercialisation to put a stop to surrogacy-for-profit. No doubt in part because it was an American initiative, undertaken during a period of resistance to the 'Americanisation' of Britain under Thatcher, surrogacy remains much more limited in Britain than it is in the United States and many other countries.

The public was also divided in relation to abortion. Although public opinion surveys in Britain indicate growing acceptance of abortion in the 1980s, which is permitted by law under specific conditions, it remains a contentious issue. Although even 79 per cent of Catholics in Britain, for example, support a woman's right to abortion in cases of rape or grave threat to the mother's health, acceptance is generally less widespread in relation to more 'preferential' reasons to terminate a pregnancy, such as financial, relational or other circumstantial concerns (although even for these criteria a slight majority supports a woman's right to choose, see figures in Harding 1988: 41). Much less widely accepted is the provision of contraception or contraceptive advice to minors under the age of sixteen (60 per cent against and 30 per cent in favour, Harding 1988: 40).

One of the reasons the Thatcher government was so reluctant to move forward quickly on the human fertilisation and embryology legislation, in spite of urgent appeals by the legal, medical and scientific communities to do so, was the inevitable political penalty for this process. In matters as contentious and volatile as reproductive politics, governments often seek to avoid the inevitable alienation of one constituency or another in this area of limited compromise measures. Sure enough, the debate about human fertilisation and embryology in Britain quickly became embroiled in the abortion controversy.[16] In 1985, parliamentary member Enoch Powell introduced the Unborn Children (Protection) Bill, based on a Right-to-Life argument that life begins at conception. Included in his effort to ban abortion was also a bid to ban embryo research, and the use of embryo transfer in IVF. In so far as IVF inevitably involves the production of some embryos that are not used, so-called 'spare' embryos, and also relies on embryo research to improve its success rates, Powell and his supporters sought to outlaw such techniques. The unanticipated amount of support for the Powell Bill, and its linking of assisted conception technologies and embryo research to abortion so disturbed the scientific community that they quickly established a lobby group, PROGRESS, to argue their case and retrieve public support.

During parliamentary debate of the Human Fertilisation and Embryology Act, in both the House of Lords and the House of Commons, over the full course of the 1989–90 session, the issues of abortion and of embryo research again emerged as the most contentious topics. Special time for debate was allocated for both matters. On the matter of abortion, legislative changes were made to lower the upper time limit for abortion, through widening the criteria for 'late' abortions. In terms of embryo research, agreement was reached that it should be allowed to proceed in the interests of improving human reproductive and genetic health, and contributing to basic science. However, it would be restricted to a period of fourteen days after fertilisation, and be subject to regulation in the form of a licensing body. I return to some of these provisions in more detail in the conclusion.

Britain's Human Fertilisation and Embryology Act remains the most comprehensive legislation on assisted conception, and related techniques, anywhere in the world. Only Canada has engaged in a public debate of similar proportions, although less comprehensive measures have been debated in many countries. Each of these debates, in Germany, Australia, France, Denmark (to name but a few) and most recently the United States, reveals a cultural specificity to contestation over juridical control of 'the facts of life'. In each context, as in the 'virgin birth' debates, the precise details of fertilisation and embryology – in short, conception theories, become the focus of passionate campaigns from a wide sector of the population, not only including doctors, scientists and religious leaders, but families with genetic disease, infertility support organisations, disability rights groups, feminist coalitions, and a wide range of other parties. For the anthropologist, the public record of these debates, and their rootedness in specific perspectives, offer an intriguing replay of some of the oldest debates in social theory, as Ginsburg's study has so powerfully shown (1989). In turn, one of the major arguments supporting the approach taken in this book is simply the enormous amount of material available on which to base similar, comparative studies of these debates in international perspective, each one in turn offering refractions on the cultural history of social theory as well as the scope of contemporary cultural diversity.

POPULAR REPRESENTATIONS OF ASSISTED CONCEPTION

I have written elsewhere on the popular media representation of assisted conception in England in the late 1980s (Franklin 1990), and in particular of the idiom of 'desperateness' which so often was used to characterise the quest for conception of infertile women and couples (see also Pfeffer 1987). While I do not wish to rehearse that argument in detail here, a few points are worth repeating in the interests of contextualisation. It should be noted that beginning with the birth of Louise Brown, which received worldwide media attention in the summer of 1978, conception narratives derivative of the world of achieved conception have provided a steady supply of late twentieth century procreation stories (see also Franklin and McNeil 1993). A compilation of such accounts, modelled on Montagu's famous catalogue of Australian conception accounts (1937) could likewise be entitled *Coming Into Being Among the Euro-Americans*. In England, popular media accounts of assisted conception were distinctively formulaic in their narrative structure, combining established generic and sequential conventions to organise a telling tale of missed conceptions. These media accounts were accompanied by a flurry of popular handbooks and guidebooks to the world of achieved conception. Since these were among the most important means by which a wider public became acquainted with the new reproductive technologies, they offer an important perspective on the changing cultural meanings mobilised in and through conception stories. In the account below, I draw on only some of these accounts to explore certain key features of popular representations of infertility.

The following is an extract from the Sunday edition of the London *Times*, depicting what ubiquitously came to be known as the 'desperate' infertile couple. It is an extract that is highly characteristic of the public representation of the encounter between failed conjugal reproductive potential and newfound medical-scientific means of salvation, namely in vitro fertilisation and other assisted conception techniques. Importantly, this extract is organised as an evocative narrative, and in its composition articulates the core, indeed formulaic, features of the myriad such representations in the English press during the 1980s.

> The bright clusters of snapshots pinned to the memo board in a London clinic are a constant reminder that at least some dreams come true. Every picture of a new-born baby tells its own story of a successful fight against infertility. More than anything else, Tessa Horton wants to add to that collection. But she is 38 now and after five years of disappointment, she knows the odds are against her. Neither she nor her husband Michael will surrender their dream while the doctors continue to offer them even a slender hope ... For the Hortons and an estimated one million other couples in Britain striving to overcome childlessness, doctors can now resort to a remarkable and increasing number of treatments. Advances in the use of drugs, surgical techniques and in vitro

fertilisation mean that babies are now being born to couples who until quite recently would have been described as hopeless cases.

(Prentice, *The Sunday Times* 1986: 10)

Most evident in this account is the gap between hope for success and means of fulfilment. It could be described as an account which celebrates the potential union between a natural desire for a biological family, and the ability of natural science to provide one. As a narrative, this account makes evident the popular appeal of IVF, according to a logic of biological science in the service of a biological family. Importantly, it is a narrative of hope: hope for children via scientific progress. This is a narrative about trying to conceive against the odds, with the help of state-of-the-art technology. As such, it is a narrative that foregrounds the ambiguity and contingency of conception, rather than its certainty. Finally, as a narrative, it conforms generically both to the conventions of romance, in providing an obstacle to be overcome, as well as the conventions of heroism, by depicting scientific pioneers on the verge of a breakthrough.[17]

Important to such accounts is the representation of the losses suffered by infertile couples because of their failure to conceive. The *Warnock Report* also emphasised a loss of social identity, specifically a sense of belonging:

Childlessness can be a source of stress even to those who have deliberately chosen it . . . They may feel that they will be unable to fulfill their own or other peoples' expectations. They may feel excluded from a whole range of human activity and particularly the activities of their childrearing contemporaries.

(Warnock 1985: 9)

The need for social approval is thus one of the important losses creating the 'desperateness' of the infertile couple. This view is also expressed in a popular infertility guidebook written by a doctor:

For most individuals, life moves in a progression that is highlighted by the events of marriage and childbirth. When this progression is interrupted by infertility, it produces an effect beyond just the physical absence of a child. A couple may, for the first time, feel they have lost control over a significant part of their lives. Their own anxieties about infertility may be magnified by well-meaning, but unthinking, relatives and friends who continually ask about the prospects of pregnancy.

(Glass 1984: 1)

It is because life moves in a progression that infertility poses an obstacle to happiness. It is the disruption of the normal progression in the lives of 'most individuals' which causes them to 'feel they have lost control' and to suffer from 'anxieties' about their infertility. Socially and emotionally, the stress of childlessness is attributed to failure in fulfilling conventional adult roles and failure to 'found a family'. The cause of 'desperateness', in other words, is represented as a failure to conform to social norms.

In addition to social pressures, many popular representations of infertility also draw on the idea that there are natural, biological or genetic pressures to have children which cannot be suppressed. The opening paragraph of *The Infertility Handbook*, written by a doctor and a science journalist, expresses this view:

> Call it a cosmic spark or spiritual fulfilment, biological need or human destiny – the desire for a family rises unbidden from our genetic souls. In centuries past, to multiply was to prevail – the family was stronger, and better able to survive than the individual.
>
> (Bellina and Wilson 1986: xv)

The conflation of the language of evolutionary genetics with that of spiritual desire and personal fulfilment in this passage (e.g: 'genetic souls') is revealing. It suggests that the desire to have a family is not merely social, but primordial. It is represented as being genetically determined by our evolutionary heritage and essential to our survival both as individuals and as a species.

Such views were often expressed publicly by assisted conception professionals, such as the late Patrick Steptoe, who believed 'it is a fact that there is a biological drive to reproduce' and that 'women who deny this drive, or in whom it is frustrated, show disturbances in other ways' (quoted in Stanworth 1987: 15). Similarly, the *Warnock Report* claimed that:

> In addition to social pressures to have children there is, for many, a powerful urge to perpetuate their genes through a new generation. This desire cannot be assuaged by adoption.
>
> (Warnock 1985: 9)

The representation of a powerful genetic drive to reproduce, coupled with the influence of social pressures, establishes the 'social and natural facts' of infertility, much as this dichotomy structured earlier accounts of kinship, family and procreation in anthropology. The view that the urge to found a family has evolutionary significance,

and derives from a primordial human desire, also recalls the importance of such arguments to turn-of-the-century debates about the
origins of sociality, the beginnings of the pair bond, and the
regulation of sexuality and marriage. The model of society being, in
this sense, 'after nature' is clearly evident in these accounts, as they
are in the myriad others of which these are typical. This connection,
however, takes an interesting turn in relation to the introduction of
new technology.

If 'the desire to found a family' is a primordial drive that 'rises
unbidden from our genetic souls', then 'life's progression' from
marriage to childbirth is not merely a social convention, but part of
the flow of life itself. It is, in this sense, a naturalised progression.
However, this natural sequence of events has also to take a particular
social form. It is implicit in the account of couples 'feeling excluded
from a whole range of activities' and experiencing a loss of 'the kind
of life they would have led' in order to 'fulfil their own or other
peoples' expectations' that the desire is to conform to established
social conventions. When Patrick Steptoe argues that it is a 'biological
fact' that women possess a 'biological drive to reproduce', he is not
concerned with lesbian or single women, whose exclusion from
conventional social arrangements may lessen the likelihood of their
having children. To the contrary, he firmly opposed such women
having children at all, on the grounds that it is unnatural and morally
wrong. In this sense, the social conventions are also naturalised, in the
sense of being 'modelled on', or 'rooted in' or 'determined by' nature.

Reproduction is, of course, a highly naturalised activity in the
Euro-American cultural tradition. Into this highly naturalised
domain, then, enters medical science, on behalf of the 'desperate'
infertile couples for whom 'life's progression' has been held hostage
to the random injustice of nature's lottery in making them unable to
conceive. This is the critical link in popular media representations,
such as the one described earlier, through which the 'desperate'
desire for a child provides the lead-in to the 'medical hope for a
cure'. In the same account quoted earlier from the *Sunday Times*, it
is asserted that:

> *Their only hope* lies with the gynaecologists, andrologists, ur-
> ologists, endocrinologists and others who specialise in treating
> infertility, including the growing number of experts in in vitro
> fertilisation – the so called 'test-tube baby' doctors.
>
> (Prentice 1986: 10, emphasis added)

Thus, within and framed by the hopes and desires of the 'desperate' infertile couple (or, in this case, the 'desperate' infertile woman 'Tessa Horton'), is a description of the latest techniques and procedures being developed by state-of-the-art clinicians and researchers to overcome the obstacle of infertility. The article continues:

> Some surgeons are now applying lasers to tubal surgery. Mr Simon Wood, a consultant gynaecologist at the Royal Devon and Exeter Hospital, has achieved a 33 per cent live birth rate in a small number of patients using a laser. . . . Last November, Australian scientists announced they were the first team to successfully freeze human ova. . . . Professor David Baird is trying to develop tests to identify which fertilised human eggs are healthy and which are abnormal. They hope to exclude abnormal 'pre-embryos' from IVF treatment.
>
> (Prentice 1986: 10)

A similar emphasis upon the 'hope' that bridges a biological inability to conceive and the newfound capacity of biological science to provide solutions is emphasised in *Miracle Babies and Other Happy Endings* written by a fertility specialist:

> Only a few years ago most couples with infertility problems had to turn to adoption or remain childless. But now, with advances in pharmaceuticals, micro-surgery, in vitro fertilisation and embryo transfer, many viable options have opened up to infertile couples – with the result that 'miracle babies' are being born every day. *There is every reason for hope.*
>
> (Perloe 1986: ix, original emphasis)

The *Warnock Report* also offered a similar version of scientific progress, describing the development of in vitro fertilisation as 'a considerable achievement' which 'opened up new horizons in the alleviation of infertility'. In their Report, the Committee claimed that advances in embryology created 'hope of remedying defective embryos' creating 'pride in technological achievement' and thus 'pleasure at the new found means to relieve . . . the unhappiness of infertility' (Warnock 1985: 4).

These positive assessments of natural science in the service of the natural family comprise an extension of being, as Strathern describes it, 'after nature' (1992a). In the same way social conventions build upon a natural foundation, so too does technology, as a social achievement, extend nature's purpose. Representationally, that is, in terms of narrative structure, it is significant that the depiction of scientific achievements in the form of new techniques are inserted within the narrative sequence framed by the hopes and desires of infertile couples. Where 'life's progression' breaks off for infertile couples, their losses open up a space into which science and technology are positioned as a bridge, much as IVF was initially used to 'bridge the gaps' in conception caused by blocked Fallopian tubes. The embedding of a technological sequence within the larger sequence of 'life's progression' helps naturalise the technology itself as 'giving nature a helping hand'.

The frame of 'life's progression' is restored by forms of narrative closure characteristic of the coverage given to successful couples. Needless to say, little coverage was provided of the majority of couples who failed to progress successfully through IVF to the desired outcome of a 'take-home baby'.[18] Complementing the emphasis on hope is the language of miracles consistently used to describe success in the context of assisted conception.

Some examples from local newspapers in the 1980s illustrate this form of narrative closure. In one such article, the paper ran a front page story of a successful couple, parents of triplets, beneath the banner headline: 'OUR GORGEOUS TINY WONDERS'. Above the headline are photographs of all three infants (attached to life support). The couple are prominently pictured below, with the caption 'Delighted parents Mandy and Clint Baker overjoyed by their instant family.' At the end of the article, it is noted that 'the couple met at a [city] Kissogram agency where Mandy worked when Clint joined as a "gorilla-gram". Now he runs his own garage and says they will have to move from their two-bedroomed semi into a bigger house' (Matthews and Jones 1987: 1).

A second article, entitled TEST-TUBE BABY FOR THRILLED PARENTS, also received front page coverage in the *Daily News* (29 March 1988). Described as a 'miracle of modern science' and as a 'triumph for the team who pioneered [the city's] IVF programme', 'test-tube baby Samuel' is featured in the requisite photograph of the happy couple with their longed-for progeny. In the accompanying text readers learn that:

> Proud parents Phil and Carol Goulding last night trembled with joy as they cradled their newborn son, Samuel. . . . For Carol and Phil . . . 9lb 5oz Samuel is nothing less than a miracle. 'We've been married 14 years and trying for a baby for 12', said 37-year

old Carol. 'I still can't believe he's finally here.' Carol began treatment in 1977 ... and almost gave up hope of ever having a child when an operation to unblock her Fallopian tubes failed. ... 'We were on holiday in Scotland when I realised I was pregnant, and we were just so happy.'

(Cunningham 1988: 1)

These personal details perform an important function in providing narrative closure. Their presence indicates the need for more than a medical 'solution' to the problem of infertility. Through details about their jobs, houses, holidays and happiness, these accounts not only provide a 'good story', but they do so through creating a traditional happy ending, which re-establishes the couple within the conventions of heterosexual romance, confirming the unity of the conjugal and the procreative function, buttressed by references to upward mobility, social approval and establishment through becoming a family. The themes of hope, fulfilment and 'dreams come true' are thus linked to the 'miracle of modern science', a 'test-tube baby'. Hence, as the 'desperate' infertile couple narrative begins by describing the emotional desires of the would-be parents, so it also closes by referring back to their emotions and fulfilment, thereby enclosing the interior narrative of scientific progress within a frame of reference to heterosexual reproductive desire and the maintenance of established social conventions.

In a sense, then, the 'desperate' infertile couple narratives 'embody' or enclose scientific process by re-embedding it within familiar, recognisable details of ordinary, everyday life. The point is that this containment of the potentially quite disruptive or troubling implications of a 'test-tube baby' is evident in the very structure of these narratives. This is very characteristic of *popular* narrative, which works by inviting identification and then rewarding, or 'satisfying' it. The narrative tension, provided by an 'obstacle' to fulfilment is overcome, followed by celebratory closure. It is significant that the 'happy couples' stories present both a continuity and a commensurability between biological science and the biological family. The achieved route of conception stands in for conjugality and family as *social* achievements, 'after nature', though in this context, 'after technology' as well. In sum, it is the substitutability of natural, social and technological 'facts' these narratives demonstrate which indexes particular features of the kinship universe within which they are operative, and of which they are also transformative.

Together, then, these elements of the achieved conception success story articulate core features of both the 'enterprise culture' context in which they are produced, and the wider set of cultural values attached to conjugality, procreativity and family in English society. As purchasers of private healthcare services, couples 'buy in' to the 'dream come true' of a family of their own. In turn, they sell their two-bedroomed semi to purchase a larger home. Through these means they become established, and are enabled to realise the way of life they had imagined for themselves, before 'life's progression' was brought unexpectedly to an impasse. As self-reliant individuals, seeking to extend conjugality into family and home-ownership, they express a desire for social achievement through biological reproduction. Assisted conception, in these representations, precisely reproduces the core analogies of English kinship, just as it also fulfils the promise of the enterprise culture in the form of widened consumer choice through market deregulation and expansion.

The language of hope, miracles and progress are also significant features of these accounts. 'Hope' is the important flip-side of the fact that assisted conception usually does not work. This has important implications for the next three chapters, where it is explored in greater depth. 'Progress' is like 'hope' in this respect, for it signals the continuing effort to overcome obstacles, to transcend limits and to explore new horizons. 'Progress' also importantly signifies the desire for improvement, which is what society also imposes on the 'nature' it is 'rooted in' or 'based upon'. Assisted conception is to reproduction what progress is to nature: it is a 'helping hand' assisting nature to progress as it was meant to do. Likewise, assisted conception is to reproduction what enterprise is to the national economy – a vital force for change, improvement and achievement.

At the same time, the neat symmetry of the 'dominant' cultural logic valorising assisted conception is somewhat contradicted by the language of 'miracles.' To begin with, the miracle is both 'of modern science' and of nature. The miracle baby both attests to the miraculous powers of science and to the miracle of new life, that is, of nature. In so far as the 'miracle' is of modern science, it is no longer 'after nature', but displacing it; technology also 'does service for' ideas of the natural. The 'helping hand' is more like a corporate takeover, through which the agency of technology becomes dominant, not merely 'assisting' conception but literally removing it from the body altogether. It is the disembodiment of conception that effects this shift, through which the 'facts of life' are not only relocated to the Petri dish, but subject to retemporalisation, through cryo-preservation, and redirection through modification and alteration. This 'assistance' has various consequences of displacement which are discussed in more depth in the conclusion. Here, I wish to conclude this section through a brief consideration of the formula of natural science in the service of the natural family which so thoroughly characterises the representation of assisted conception as 'giving nature a helping hand'.

ENGLISHNESS AND IDEAS OF THE NATURAL

As noted in the final section of the last chapter, the naturalisation of reproduction has become the focus of increasing attention in the theorisation of kinship and gender. As part of the effort to 'de-naturalise' the 'facts of life,' it is important to attend closely to the contradictory dimensions of ideas of the natural. Not only are constructions of the natural culturally and historically specific; they are also shifting and contradictory. As is the case in the analysis of science, a cultural domain to which ideas of the natural are central, it is important not to overstate the discursive or cultural determinism operative in the 'naturalising' process.

None the less, attention to the role of ideas of the natural as a significant domain of Euro-American cultural production has become increasingly central to social and cultural theory.[19] As MacNaghten and Urry argue in their attempt to outline a sociology of nature:

Until very recently [an] academic division between a world of social facts and a world of natural facts was largely uncontentious. . . . [O]nce it is acknowledged that ideas of nature [are] fundamentally intertwined with dominant ideas of society, we have then to address what ideas of society have been reproduced, legitimated, excluded, validated, etc. through appeals to nature or the natural.

(MacNaghten and Urry 1995: 204, 208)

As noted earlier, Raymond Williams was among the first to investigate the significance of ideas of the natural within a specifically English tradition. He argues that a separate domain of the natural emerges in conjunction with early eighteenth-century natural scientific conceptions of nature as a material world governed by law and order. Lawlike mechanical nature is both personified and unified within European science, paralleling the Judaeo-Christian model of a deity that is also singular, personified and originary. In Williams's view, Nature replaces, though complements, God as an origin of the diversity of life, including Man, with the advent of Darwinism. For Strathern, the formation of a domain of the social which is seen to come 'after nature' stems, in part, from the Darwinian model of genealogy. Hence, she argues, humanity comes to be seen as both descended from and consanguinous with nature, at the same time that human society comes to be seen as modelled on a departure from the state of nature through the invention of social laws. This is precisely the question that so preoccupied early European social theorists, whose concern with origins was exhaustive. The preservation of the 'after nature' model of society, as both part of and distinct from the order of nature, is evident in the hybrid institution of kinship, as composed of 'social and natural facts'. As MacNaghten and Urry point out, it is only recently that this longstanding convention of assuming a given distinction between the natural and the social has been made explicit. Strathern's concern is with the literalisation that ensues from the 'making explicit' of the nature/ society, or nature/ culture opposition. For sociologists such as MacNaghten and Urry, a similar 'flattening' effect to that described by Strathern is evident at the level of 'reflexive modernisation', referring to an increased consciousness of 'nature' as being in need of 'assistance'.[20]

Cultural historians in Britain have long been attentive to the importance of 'languages of nature' in the formation of both English and British national culture (Jordanova 1986). The importance of the debate surrounding the rise of Darwinian models of evolution has been a particularly important strand in this tradition of historical study (Young 1973; Beer 1983). Analysis of the historical constitution of ideas of the natural, and of 'life itself' also figure centrally in the work of Foucault, who has been attentive to their reinscription through the modern biological sciences (1971). The significance of cross-overs between literary and scientific representation have figured prominently in much scholarship addressing the importance of ideas of the natural to a specifically English national identity (McNeil 1987). However, as both Strathern (1992a) and Bouquet (1993) have demonstrated, these formations can also be traced in relation to both the history of social theory and the constitution of certain features of social organisation, in particular of kinship.

In a fascinating study of the relationship between literary and scientific representations of reproductive technology in early twentieth-century England, Susan Squier documents the enormous fascination with the image of 'babies in bottles' well before the advent of assisted conception several decades later. As her account makes clear, the vision of natural science as a means of implementing social progress through a redesign of reproductive processes is not a recent innovation. It is, however, in some ways arguably a distinctively English fascination. In describing, for example, how the young Julian Huxley was influenced by the Victorian children's story *The Water Babies.* written by Charles Kingsley (1863), Squier suggests that evolutionary analogies deeply permeated understandings of morality, society and the individual (1994: 294). Tracing the chain of analogies occasioning what Strathern describes as 'Darwin's loan' (of kinship to describe nature as a unified system), Squier argues that evolutionary ideas became a powerful idiom of progress and improvement of society through control of reproduction (see also Beer 1983).

As Yanagisako and Delaney point out, the importance of the belief in progress to the construction of nature as a competitive field of 'survival of the fittest' was explicitly noted by Marx in his assessment of Darwinism: 'Darwin recognizes among beasts and plants his English society with its divisions of labor, competition, opening of new markets, "inventions" and the Malthusian "struggle for existence"' (cited in Yanagisako and Delaney 1995: 5). As it became possible to look to 'nature' for explanations of human society and character, so too was Darwin's loan 'read back', as Strathern describes it, enabling nature to become subject to visions of social improvement. This traffic is in many ways distinctively British. Much as it has informed the Euro-American imagination more broadly, it has specific roots in England where the national culture has long been formed in relation to the zig-zagging repeat of analogies linking nature, progress and society.

The realm of new reproductive technologies is, therefore, an important context through which to connect the historic importance of ideas of the natural, and the cultural value accorded scientific progress, in the formation of English cultural identity as well as in the effort to understand processes of naturalisation more broadly. As with any project concerned with broad, overarching cultural symbols, values and concepts, exploration of their significance is usefully explored through concrete empirical study of their social articulation. The next three chapters present one perspective of this sort, at the point of encounter between nature, technology and choice occasioned by the advent of assisted conception. In the conception narratives derivative of this encounter become clear both the power and the ambiguity of symbols and values often rendered more coherently from a distance. Close up, the 'biological facts' of reproduction themselves become complex signifiers of both change and continuity in the context of their technological instrumentalisation. The dilemmas and hopes expressed in the pursuit of a miracle baby, and the complex negotiations occasioning the encounter with high-tech conceptive success and failure, illustrate both the intensity and the distinctiveness of what it means literally to embody scientific progress as an expression of reproductive desire and consumer choice.

Chapter 3

The 'obstacle course': the reproductive work of IVF

It just takes over, there's no doubt about it.

(Jeanette Ives)

INTRODUCTION

In this and the subsequent three chapters, women's experience of IVF is investigated in terms of how women undergoing the procedure describe the experience of IVF as 'a way of life'. This perspective is informed by the phrase I encountered frequently during interviews, of 'Living IVF'. Conveyed by this expression is the sense of how IVF 'takes over' a woman's life, as is also expressed in the headnote to this chapter. I argue an ethnographic approach to IVF is one way to approach this intensity, in terms of how it is generated by various aspects of the technique. Although the accounts presented here can in no way be considered representative in a sociological sense, they are indicative of the way in which the experience of IVF is lived and embodied, and how this experience is described and narrated.

As with any ethnographic project, designed to elicit key terms or phrases through which people describe their own experience, certain condensed nodes of meaning emerge in descriptions of achieved conception. These can be considered points where several layers of meaning converge to produce an overdetermined effect. They are often to be found in phrases that are heard again and again across a range of different contexts and from a number of different sources. In re-analysing the interview material and fieldnotes, I discovered a number of phrases of this sort, which I then used to rework, organise and present the material.

Hence, this chapter is entitled 'The "obstacle course"', which is another phrase often used to describe the experience of undergoing IVF. The headnote describes the way in which IVF 'takes over', which was another, related phrase that came up again and again. Both terms have the kind of overdetermined status which makes them useful for explicating a wide range of features of the IVF experience. In this chapter, then, the obstacle course metaphor is used to present the various stages of IVF and the physical, emotional and psychological difficulties they pose. These in turn explain why IVF 'takes over', and illustrate concretely what this expression means. A sub-theme of the chapter is indicated by its subtitle, 'the reproductive work of IVF'.[1] This too provides a connecting thread, albeit an analytic one, linking a range of different features of the IVF experience, which, it is suggested here, together comprise a form of reproductive labour. In the final section, the tensions between women's paid work as part of the waged labour force is compared with their unpaid reproductive labour. This in turn provides the means for looking in another way at the most immediate demands of IVF, such as travelling, co-ordinating tasks, and general management of the 'regime' imposed by the treatment cycle.[2]

This chapter also introduces the description of IVF as a 'way of life'. The next chapter explores in more depth what is meant by this phrase, moving away from the immediate demands of treatment, to consider more broadly how IVF 'makes sense', or is made sense of, in a wider frame. The idea of a 'way of life', again, is multi-layered, referring both to IVF as a 'way of life', the lifestyles of individuals and couples, and the wider 'way of life' of the society they inhabit. Although the experience of achieved conception is not culturally bounded in a traditional anthropological sense, its description as a 'way of life' exemplifies a different kind of boundedness to this experience, providing the ethnographic frame for this research. Borrowing from cultural studies approaches to ethnography, informed by Raymond Williams's idea of 'whole ways of life' and 'whole ways of struggle', these chapters attempt to correlate the experience of 'living IVF' with broader questions about the social organisation of gender, kinship and the sexual division of labour.

Chapter 5 is entitled '"Having to try" and "Having to choose"', which are again phrases encountered often in the course of the interviews. The former statement, encountered in every interview, proved integral to the overall analysis. This statement is of particular importance because of its repeated centrality to women's descriptions of IVF. At the core of the experience of IVF is the pursuit of reproductive desire, often naturalised as an inherent human or parental drive, and therefore complicated by its realisation in the context of high technology. In such a context, the seamlessness of interplay between 'social' and 'natural' facts becomes particularly apparent. In particular, the significance of individual choice in the context of both new technology and the 'enterprise culture' of Thatcherism are discussed.

To introduce the technique of IVF, I begin with a contrast between the representation of IVF in the standard clinical introductory pamphlets, and women's descriptions of the technique. This chapter then moves on to consider the immediate physical, psychological and emotional demands of undergoing the IVF procedure. All three chapters on IVF are concerned with how women make sense of this procedure. These ways of making sense are both determined by the experience of treatment, and determining of it, as the attitudes women develop towards the procedure inform the ways in which they learn to 'manage' it, in both senses of the term.

INTRODUCING IVF: THE STANDARD IVF DESCRIPTION

The introductory descriptions of IVF distributed by the clinics involved in this study consisted of short pamphlets, compiled either by the clinics themselves or by the drug companies who produce the pharmaceuticals used in the procedure. Two primary features characterised the representation of IVF in these leaflets: IVF was always described as a 'simple' procedure, and as a 'natural' one. The simplicity of IVF was conveyed by its description as a sequence of stages or procedures: removal of the egg, in vitro fertilisation, and reimplantation of the embryo. The naturalness of the technique was emphasised through phrases such as 'giving Nature a helping hand', conveying the idea that IVF is just helping nature to do what it would have done anyway. These two representations, of IVF as simple and as natural, were combined in the image of IVF as a 'bridge', or, as one pamphlet describes it, 'a bridge to a new life'. The mechanical image of a bridge, which stands for the 'helping hand' of technology, invokes the original use of IVF to bypass blocked Fallopian tubes. In this image are united the idea of conception as a natural flow or sequence of events, and the insertion of technological assistance into a naturalised event to close the gap, as it were. The closing of the gap in turn refers also to the amelioration of the yawning gulf between reproductive desire and inability to conceive. It is the seamlessness of this transition which is the important message uniting nature, technology and reproductive desire in these accounts, as in the media accounts discussed earlier.

The following are extracts from introductory IVF pamphlets describing the technique:

> IVF involves collecting eggs from the ovary, putting them together with spermatozoa in a dish, and if those spermatozoa fertilise an egg, putting the embryo or embryos that result into the womb.
>
> (*In-Vitro Fertilization with Fertility Services*, n.d: 2)

> *In vitro* fertilisation is a technique in which the sperm and egg, instead of meeting in the fallopian tube, are made to meet literally 'in glass' – i.e. the test tube (or a dish).
>
> (Information Booklet: *In Vitro Fertilization and GIFT*, Infertility Advisory Centre, n.d.: 3)

> IVF or (IVF-ET) entails bringing the male sperm and the female egg together outside the body, so that fertilisation occurs. The tiny fertilised egg (now called an embryo) is then transferred back to the womb to develop normally.
>
> (*In-Vitro Fertilisation: Some Questions Answered*, Serono Laboratories (UK) Ltd, n.d.: 1)

> Since 1978, *in vitro* fertilisation has provided a positive solution to many couples' infertility. The principle is simple: the function of the defective fallopian tubes is assumed artificially under strict conditions in the laboratory. This takes scarcely 48 hours.
>
> (*When Nature Fails . . . A Modern View of In Vitro Fertilization*, Organon, n.d.: 27)

> Commonly referred to as the test-tube baby technique, IVF is the technique of mixing the woman's eggs (ova) with sperm from her partner in a small dish or test tube in the laboratory, to allow fertilisation to occur. Once the ova are fertilised and have divided, one or more of the fertilised eggs (pre-embryos) are replaced into the woman's uterus through the cervix.
>
> (*Fertility Services*, AMI Healthcare, n.d.: 2)

While technically accurate, descriptions such as these, which emphasise the simplicity of IVF treatment, fail to convey several important aspects of the procedure. For one, they fail to convey the amount of procedure involved in removal of eggs. For another, they do not convey the number of ways in which the procedure can fail, or, in IVF parlance, lead to the cycle being 'abandoned'. The conflation of technology and nature in these accounts is partly facilitated by the simultaneous conflation of 'IVF', the actual point at which the egg is fertilised in vitro, with the entire process of 'IVF', which involves much more than that. Finally, the naming of the technique as 'IVF', for the one component of it which occurs independently from a woman's body, precisely emphasises its technological dimension, very much in contrast to the way this is de-emphasised by describing it as 'natural'.

Other aspects of these representations of IVF are also notable. For example, they describe no agents. Or, it might be said the only agency in evidence is the 'invisible hand' of technology. Techno-scientific agency is consequently naturalised, as a force in and of itself: 'the function . . . is assumed . . . by the laboratory'. Conception here takes place through a union of technological and natural processes, consistently represented in the passive voice. The technique of IVF is positioned as a helpmate to nature: it 'allow[s] fertilisation to occur'. In so far as Euro-Americans imagine kinship as the 'social construction of natural facts', IVF is here described as materialising that equation: the natural facts of conception, the meeting of the egg and sperm, are facilitated by the 'helping hand' of technology. Conception is literally pieced together. Yet, this is no ordinary construction process. The building blocks are those of life itself. Hence, in so far as the unfolding of 'the facts of life' are both narrativised and naturalised as the biological sequence through which Euro-Americans understand coming into being, these representations of IVF embed technology into nature in a manner that makes perfect sense of this contradiction.

WOMEN'S DESCRIPTIONS OF IVF: THE 'OBSTACLE COURSE'

A useful contrast can be drawn between the preceding introductory accounts of IVF and a description of it by one of the women interviewed. As Kate Quigley[3] describes her experience:

Um, on the first day of the cycle, the first day of my period, we start with a, I have a nasal spray, which I use four times a day, one spray up each nostril, and then I had, then you have I think they are steroids, somebody said they were steroids, and then you take two in the morning and one at night, that's two, to help to grow healthy eggs. On the fourth day of your cycle you start with

Perganol injections and my GP gave those to me, so I just had to go up to the surgery and he did those for me. And also on the fourth day you have to collect your urine and collect for twenty-four hours and then you have to send a sample off so that they can measure your oestrogen that's in your urine so they can see what response your body is making to all the drugs. And then on the sixth day you go for the first scan, that's when they can see if any eggs are growing and how many. You go for a scan every other day, and then on both occasions they said that on the 11th day, they said that the eggs, the follicles were sort of large enough for me to be given the hCG injection which they give about thirty-five hours before they aspirate the eggs, the hCG injection, it makes you ovulate, because without that you wouldn't ovulate. And then thirty-five hours later you have the eggs aspirated and if they fertilise and divide then two days later you put the embryos back.

Noticeably, this account puts most emphasis on the process of ovulation induction, and least on the actual process of IVF, which is in fact not even mentioned. From the point of view of a woman who has experienced IVF, in other words, the technique is defined *most* by what is missing from the introductory descriptions, and *least* by what is actually in them.

Far from being described as a simple technique, women repeatedly described the unanticipated complexity of the IVF procedure. Even if they were well acquainted with the range of techniques involved, they were often unprepared for the extent to which the technique 'took over' their lives through its considerable demands upon them. As Jeanette Ives, who is quoted in the headnote to this chapter, put it:

It's a very intense procedure and if you're up at the hospital every day virtually and you are being monitored all the time so obviously it's a very intense time and you do get very involved in it all. Much more so than you imagine you will do, it's not like having one injection, you know, it's really involved. . . . And it does sort of take over your life to quite a big extent.

In addition to finding the technique more complicated than expected, and suprisingly 'intense', the number of things that could go wrong during the cycle was not anticipated accurately. This too can be seen as a result of the difference between IVF as a clinical procedure and IVF from a woman's point of view. A frequent way in which this discovery was represented was in terms of a series of hurdles or stages: an obstacle race. The analogy of the obstacle race was for many women the most effective way to describe their experience of the actual procedure of IVF.

Descriptions of IVF as an obstacle race or a set of hurdles to be overcome were very common. Several women used this analogy to describe their experience of the technique:

It's like, to me, when I think about it, it's like running the Grand National without a horse and with your legs tied together and with a blindfold on. I don't know how long the Grand National is . . . it feels like that . . . but with all the brooks and everything else, and you've got to get over every single hurdle and you can still fall at the finish line.

(Meg Flowers)

And you think the first time, oh yes, it's going to work, even though they say the first time doesn't usually work . . . and the reason the disappointment is stronger than you'd expect is because it's like a set of hurdles, and each one that you're successful you build your hope a bit more.

(Karen Clarke)

Well, just reading in an article and coming to the treatment I didn't realise that there were so many obstacles that you've got to get over, you've got to get over each obstacle one at a time before you can carry on to the next, you know there may be a problem where you just don't ovulate for one reason or another, so that cycle has to be abandoned, and then try again the next cycle and then the problem is whether they fertilise, and then the problem of whether they will divide.

(Susan Doyle)

Far from describing a simple technique, these descriptions address the difference between IVF in theory and IVF in practice. In theory, each stage leads to the next stage, but in practice each stage becomes a potential source of failure, and thus an 'obstacle'. In descriptions such as these, the emphasis is not only on the unexpected difficulties encountered, but on the high risk of failure at each stage, a fact for which most women, despite being well informed beforehand, were emotionally unprepared. As is also noted in the latter two descriptions, one from a woman who was a trained nurse and very knowledgeable about IVF, appreciating beforehand the high likelihood of failure, or the number of ways in which the technique can fail, is difficult both because of the reluctance not to believe it will succeed, and simply because not enough information is conveyed. These are only some of the difficulties of conveying an accurate description of what the technique involves. Ellen Brown explains how easily IVF can be underestimated:

> There's a lot more to it than you're thinking [at the outset]. As I say, it all sounds wonderful but you don't realise the small percentage that works and the lot that doesn't work. When I first went up there I was thinking oh, if there's nothing wrong with it, it's going to work. And obviously it doesn't, you know. [But] you can't help but think you are going to be one of the successful ones, and that if nothing goes wrong you are going to get pregnant.

There is both an initial reluctance not to believe 'you are going to be one of the successful ones'[4] and an underestimation of the number of things that can go wrong during the cycle.

Yet another consequence of the obstacle race element in the experience of IVF is its impact on definitions of success and failure. Initially, women define success and failure simply in terms of whether the technique results in a 'take home baby', the ultimate success of IVF. This changes as the obstacle race element of the technique comes to be better appreciated. Coming to see IVF as a series of hurdles has the effect of a treatment being seen as successful if it progresses beyond some of these obstacles, *even if it later fails*. But failure is also much harder to accept the further along the cycle it comes. Failure is absolute, and is described as 'the cycle being abandoned' or, simply, 'abandonment'. Success, on the other hand, is measured in terms of degrees of success, or relative success, more often than in terms of complete success, which is the exception.[5]

To appreciate more fully the series of stages or hurdles involved in IVF, a schematic representation of the serial components of the procedure is provided below. This sequence also includes a brief indication of the demands of the technique in terms of the work that is required at each stage.

The stages of IVF

1 Previous infertility investigations diagnosing, or not, source of obstacle to conception (if necessary).

2 Choosing an IVF programme (investigation, selection, referral, initial consultation, admission onto programme).

3 Initial work-up (updating of infertility tests, etc.).

4 Preparation for first cycle (getting drugs from GP, arranging time off work, arranging transport, financial arrangements, etc.).

5 Ovulation induction (two- to three-week period of daily injections, tablets, hormonal nasal spray, ultra-sound scans, urine collection and sampling, blood tests).

6 Egg aspiration (hCG (human chorionic gonadotrophin) injection thirty-five hours before removal of eggs, valium/pethadine twelve hours beforehand, aspiration – surgical removal of up to thirty ova (general anaesthetic in some cases)).

7 Embryo transfer (ET) (if eggs have fertilised and divided successfully, up to three are selected and transferred into the cervix through a catheter after twenty-four to forty-eight hours).

8 Pregnancy testing (following a two-week waiting period, blood tests are performed to establish whether pregnancy has occurred).

9 Prenatal monitoring (if pregnancy has commenced a programme of prenatal monitoring is followed until completion of pregnancy by either miscarriage or birth). In some cases, 'selective termination' of one or more fetuses is indicated, due to a multiple pregnancy. This procedure is, however, controversial and is not widely used.[6]

10 Birth (when they continue to term, IVF pregnancies are more likely to involve caesarian section, and are also more likely to result in pre-mature birth and congenital abnormality, due to the higher incidence of multiple pregnancies).

Again, as is evident from this list, in vitro fertilisation itself is one of the few aspects of treatment in which neither the woman nor her partner are involved. It is also notable that this stage, for which the technique is named, occurs well along in the cycle and is not always achieved by couples undergoing treatment. During the first two weeks of treatment, the main aim is to induce successful ovulation. Successful egg maturation must then be followed by successful egg removal. The ova must then fertilise and divide. Finally, the fertilised ova must successfully implant in the uterine lining in order for the pregnancy to 'take', and it must then continue to term in order for IVF to be a success and result in a 'take-home baby' – the bottom line of IVF success or failure.[7]

In addition to there being more potential sources of failure during an IVF programme than many women realised, it is often equally difficult to appreciate the extent to which IVF can be too 'success-ful'. In other words, if too many embryos implant, the woman may experience a multiple pregnancy. Such a prospect may not initially appear alarming, indeed it may even appear desirable to women and couples who have been trying for many years to conceive. However, even with twins there is a greater risk of perinatal complications or permanent congenital disabilities. With higher-order births of three or more, the risk factors increase considerably. In addition, even if there are no congenital or peri-natal complications, simply caring for three newborns can produce tremendous strain, effectively creating for a woman who keenly desired a baby a cruelly inverted scenario of 'overbirth', in which she finds herself in the previously un-imaginable situation of having too many babies.

In addition to being unaware of the number of stages at which the technique can fail, the obstacle race analogy is also used to describe the nature of the demands of treatment, the work involved in meeting each new stage afresh, always with an awareness of the risk of failure, yet equally with a reservoir of hope for success. All of the interviews contain references to the unanticipated demands of 'the regime', of which the following are accounts indicative:

> I think it's always easier to read about something than to actually do it. . . . But until you've experienced [IVF], you know, you say oh we do this and we collect the eggs and we do this and it all sounds quite easy.
>
> (Sylvia Newton)

> [We just thought] that it would be an administration of a drug and a recovery of an egg and then fertilisation, test-tube fertilisation, and re-implant, and essentially that *is* the procedure, but that is very much an oversimplification of the procedure.
>
> (Meg Flowers)

> I think it's more complicated than I thought it would be. . . . They just went through the basics of what exactly they did, which basically meant taking the eggs out, fertilising them outside the body, and putting them back in and that sounded quite straight-forward to me, I thought it was something you could do in an afternoon.
>
> (Mavis Norton)

In addition to being more complicated than many women initially thought, IVF is often more emotionally traumatic as well. In part, it is the unanticipated demands of treatment which make of IVF such an 'intense' experience. Likewise, it is often the first procedure that is the most overwhelming. Other factors also contribute to this sensation, however, in particular the anticipation inevitably generated at each stage of treatment, and the number of stages which must be successfully completed in order to succeed in realising 'the ultimate goal' of a take-home baby. Finally, and most obviously, there is the basic underlying stress of IVF being a woman's 'only hope' to have a child. Frances Keating, a child-minder with an adopted daughter, explains the impact of this 'last chance' quality of IVF:

> I think unless you've actually been on an IVF programme you don't really know what's involved. Because it is, I mean I must admit I went there for the IVF programme thinking you go in, you have these injections, it is all, I mean I knew it took a few days, but I didn't think it would be as traumatic as it was. I think it was the way that emotionally, the way it upset me. I found one minute I was high and the next minute I was down. Going for the injections didn't bother me, taking the tablets and all the collections, that part of it never bothered me, but it was the fact that it was my last chance, I suppose, my only hope.

The potential for failure is always, and understandably, underestimated by most women – the need to believe in the potential for success of treatment outweighing the need to recognise failure as the most likely outcome. Referring to the kinds of media accounts described in the last chapter, Meg Flowers describes how difficult it is to anticipate the number of stages at which an IVF cycle can 'go wrong':

> To say that's the procedure, which it is, sort of a, b, c, d, that's what happens, there don't seem to be that many, not as many people as I imagined actually got to the end result of even having the egg retrieved, the eggs or whatever. The insinuation seemed to be from the media I suppose that if you embark on IVF it's almost as if you are going to get there in the end, but it may take two or three times. Whereas it just seems to be incredibly more difficult than that, that almost as if the intimation is that there is definitely going to be a positive end result in it so you get from the media[8], to me, all of the positive sides of it, of the women who

are having the babies, but you don't hear an awful lot about the women who start doing tests for IVF and don't get accepted onto it or get accepted onto it and fall at different hurdles.

It is on their first cycle of IVF that women encounter most forcefully the unanticipated demands of treatment. Subsequent cycles are then undertaken with greater confidence and assurance, even satisfaction in having acquired sufficient experience to 'have a programme of it', as Patricia Evans recounts:

> The first time 'round the IVF programme itself is hard, because you don't know what you're doing. You don't know, you don't know what they're doing. You don't know, you're thinking to yourself have I got my drug regime right, have I made a mess of it, when have I got to take my next tablet, when have I got to go for my next injection, or – you're not sure what you have to do, but when you've done it once, you know, you soon remember what you have to do, and then you're thinking 'oh, I know what I have to do' and then you have a programme of it.

The repetition of certain phrases in this extract, concerning the unknown dimensions of the programme, underscores the urgency often experienced on the first cycle about 'getting it right'. Familiarity with the treatment cycle gained on the 'first time 'round' enables a greater sense of control, and the confidence required to feel 'you have a programme of it'.

The initial sense of disorientation and uncertainty is not surprising given the number of procedures to be coordinated. Again, it must be remembered both that medical matters can be more daunting than more ordinary tasks, and that there is a tremendous amount riding on a successful outcome. Both of these factors can make what would otherwise be comparatively simple tasks into an anxiety-producing test of organisational and coordinating skills.

Keeping track of the drug schedule requires integrating several courses of different hormonal preparations, including injections, tablets and nasal spray. Sara Yates, a factory worker, explains:

> You can't neglect it, you can't say like all last week you'd taken your tablets and you'd taken your spray and you think, oh, I'll leave it off tomorrow and the next, you can't do that, you've got to work it for yourself the times that you are taking it. Like me, I work mine, I take it at nine, twelve, three, six, nine, twelve, between and you know where you are, you know, you've got to

work yourself to a pattern as you know when you look at that clock, when you like three o'clock time when you are sitting there about quarter to, you know you've got another fifteen minutes and you've got to take your spray like, you know.

Learning how 'to work yourself to a pattern' requires some adjustment and can initially feel like a constant preoccupation. On later cycles, it is easier to integrate self-treatment programmes into normal daily schedules.

Many women also expressed surprise at the extent to which the programme came to dominate their lives as soon as they commenced the cycle. Pauline Harding, a doctor's wife who also worked as his secretary and looked after their young child at home, describes her busy schedule:

The only trouble is that I find is that once I start going over to the clinic, on day six of the cycle, that tends to take over. Going there, it seems to be the only thing that I think about. [My husband] will come home with loads of typing for me and I'll say 'just leave it for the moment', you know what I mean, it just sort of takes over everything. And, um . . . I don't know if that should do or not [but] it takes an hour getting there, and an hour back, and you're there for an hour and a half, it seems to take up most of the day. You come back and you're absolutely shattered. . . . As soon as you start then it seems to take over everything. I keep on thinking about the scans, and working the dates out, roughly when there will be the aspiration, and hoping that [my husband] will be able to take me, and sort of thinking, well, if it's going to be late in the afternoon I'll have to arrange for someone to have [my child], sort of trying to work out everything, I have to have everything settled in my own mind.

This is a typical description of 'women's work' in the way it describes the coordination of childcare, secretarial responsibilities and the demands of treatment having to be integrated not only on a daily basis but in the longer term. It thus presents a picture of household management which is characteristic of the ways in which several different kinds of work must be integrated, and the difficulties this can present.[9]

Both the intensity of the programme and the momentum which is generated by it were frequently commented upon aspects of the experience of IVF. In the description above, the demands of the IVF programme are described as seeming 'to take over everything'. In several interviews, IVF was similarly described as becoming a 'way of life':

> I didn't know what hit me, I honestly didn't know what hit me, I couldn't believe the intensity of the programme. . . . *All you do is eat, drink and talk IVF,* your dinner conversation revolves around how big your follicles were that day, which side you had your injection in and that sort of thing, you just do, *you just live and die IVF.*
>
> (Mary Chadwick)

> Because you go into it one hundred percent, you see, it's not something you go into half sort of. . . . You throw everything in and everything else gets pushed by, *I mean . . . you live, eat, drink – everything is IVF.* Nothing else exists . . . I wasn't interested in anything else. I felt guilty, because all I was thinking about was this like, but you can't, like it takes over everything really, because it's your chance.
>
> (Frances Keating)

In both of these descriptions, IVF is described as something you 'live, eat and drink'. It is a measure of the extent to which it is felt to 'take over' a woman's life, and the life of the entire household, that it is described in this language. That IVF becomes like the food you eat indicates the degree to which it becomes a 'way of lfe'.[10]

This feeling of 'living IVF' is similarly described in the following exchange between Sara and Kevin Yates concerning the logistics of urine collection:

H: It's something you both live, I mean it's not something you just do once. It's things like . . . I've always got a jug in a plastic bag in the car.

W: Yes, you have to take your jugs, just in case. . . . You've got to feel committed first, you've got to be prepared for that.

H: You've got to be totally dedicated. You can't go nowhere without that bloody jug in the bag, you need two or three.

W: That's it, it's become a way of life to us now, you know what I mean, I think we've got about six of these damn jugs, spread one here there and everywhere.

There is the feeling that the programme becomes inescapable, pervading every aspect of a couples' life, and requiring that they show both dedication and commitment to succeed at meeting the demands of treatment.

Part of the intensity of the programme can be explained by the amount of attention it requires to coordinate urine collection, hormone injections, travel to the clinic for scans, and so forth. There is also a forcefulness to the build-up effect of the ovulation induction period, during which egg follicles are being monitored for their rate of growth: 'I felt as if I'd gone all the way up to ninety-nine and then I've had to come all the way back down to zero again', as one woman put it. Whilst there was quite a large degree of variation in the extent to which women became involved in the technical side of IVF, a sense of having ones life taken over by the waiting, the worry, the activity and the stress was consistent. Clearly, one of the most important sources of the intensity of the programme is the potential outcome of successful treatment – a baby. This aspect of the experience of IVF, the balancing of hope for success against a realistic recognition of the likelihood of failure, was often described as a major preoccupation, and is discussed in the next chapter.

THE PHYSICAL DEMANDS OF IVF

In addition to the work of managing the various tasks involved in an IVF programme, there are also physical demands. On top of scheduling the demands of treatment into the rest of her daily routine, women have to manage their own bodies and undergo physically quite demanding procedures. This is another way in which the demands of IVF can be seen as having literally to be embodied by women undergoing the procedure. This is another way in which IVF can be seen as 'taking over' or becoming a 'way of life'.[10]

Scanning procedures

In terms of physical discomfort, many women described the scanning process as one of the most demanding aspects of the programme. The purpose of scanning with an ultrasound monitor is to evaluate the effects of the hormone injections upon the rate of follicular growth. In order for the scan to reveal a clear picture, the bladder must be full, indeed bursting. This has to be achieved in coordination with travel, and the following are typical descriptions of what many women found to be the most physically demanding component of the cycle:

Mind you, the hardest part about all this treatment is just being able to gauge your bladder right. It really is, because, honestly, you can just be right one time and another time you go, you can feel right, and you ain't got enough liquid in you. . . . And yet you can be too full for it, you can never gauge it, that's the hardest part, and some people, well, I like, you can't just let a little drop out, you know what I mean, it's ever so hard to control down there, and then you have a little top up, like you know, them are the things in with treatment, I think they are more awkward, them little things like that.

(Sara Yates)

When you are travelling every other day, then it's every day, and you have to have a full bladder, and that's discomforting in itself. You know what it is like if you are absolutely bursting, I mean I'm talking about bursting to go to the toilet, and then they are pressing something on you [the scanner], all you can think of, you are not thinking about follicles, you are just thinking 'I'm dying to go to the toilet', you know, and that's all you can think of, you see. It sounds silly, doesn't it, I don't know.

(Catharine Lewis)

A definitive feature of the ultrasound scanning procedure, then, is the requirement that women exercise physical control over a physiological process that is difficult to gauge accurately. Indeed, in conjunction with travel and the vagaries of appointment schedules characteristic of even the most well-organised clinics, 'gauging' the bladder correctly might be described as an impossible task. It is perhaps because of the standard amount of hilarity connected to anything 'down there' that such difficulties are dismissed as 'silly' in the second extract. This trivialisation of their own physical discomfort is very typical of the self-descriptions provided by many women in the study, with the exception of the aspiration procedure, as is discussed below.

The aspiration procedure

While the scans are the most demanding physical aspect of the cycle from one day to the next, the operation to remove the eggs once they have matured is the most physically traumatic single event involved in IVF. At the clinic attended by women in this study, aspiration was performed as an out-patient procedure whenever possible. This meant the avoidance of the use of general anaesthetic, which is more complicated, and was often considered undesirable by women undergoing IVF because of its after-effects. However, it is not possible to use a local anaesthetic for the entire abdominal region, and therefore women were only mildly sedated with drugs such as valium or pethadin before aspiration. As a result, women were conscious during aspiration, during which a long needle is inserted into their lower abdominal cavity to puncture the egg follicles and remove as many ova as possible with the aid of an ultrasound scanner. Anticipation of this procedure was often anxiety-producing, and an understandable amount of trepidation was often expressed concerning this component of the programme. Again, while there was some variation, with some women not finding aspiration unduly traumatic, many women described egg removal as acutely painful, as the following descriptions indicate:

I wasn't prepared for how painful the aspiration was going to be. I mean they give you a pain barrier form, and I just went off the page. . . . I don't remember anything about the aspiration at all except the pain. . . . I was in agony.

(Mary Chadwick)

I mean the first time I went and had the eggs, what do they call it, the aspiration, it bloomin' hurt and in the leaflet it said there may be some slight discomfort, but this will be perfectly bearable, and it must have been a man that wrote that, because you have a needle straight through your bladder and it does hurt, apart from the fact as well that I was wide awake. . . . And I made sure that they knew that I, you know, I was aware of what was going on and it I know it hurt. I couldn't tell you how long I was in there, and I couldn't tell you how many eggs they'd taken out. . . . Put it [the pain] extreme, it was, and especially you bear in mind you are lying there, and your bladder is full, and you can't move an inch, you know . . . you are just lying there, and I've got my nurse's hand in mine, and she must have nail ridges in her hand half an inch deep because it was, and I was crying, and all the other things I'd been through it never got to me like that!

(Mavis Norton)

They say they just put the tube in and suck out the eggs and that, and that's it, you know. . . . It was quite painful, I nearly jumped off the table.

(Jeanette Ives)

That aspiration is painful is not surprising, given that tranquillisers have no anaesthetic properties. The piercing instrument used to extract the eggs must thus be inserted while the woman is fully conscious and awake. As mentioned above, anticipation of this procedure often caused considerable anxiety, as Ruth Levy recalls:

> And if you can imagine that in your mind, you're sat there, all prepared, and you know within thirty-five hours you've got to go down there and all you know about is this needle going through your abdomen . . . and you're trying to imagine the pain before you get there, and I'm thinking 'Oh my God . . . what's it going to be like to have that needle going through my abdomen', and I couldn't come to terms with that at all, all I could think of in my mind was this big needle going through my tummy, and it wasn't going to be numbed, I was only going to be sedated slightly, but they weren't numbing it like the dentist would do . . . and I thought, 'God, that needle's going to go through my tummy', and I'm looking at my tummy thinking 'where's that needle going to go through', because I just could not imagine it.

Exceptionally, women do not find the aspiration excrutiatingly painful. Jennifer Young, who was, perhaps significantly, pregnant as a result of IVF at the time of the interview, even described it as enjoyable:

> I actually rather enjoyed the aspiration, I mean everybody was saying wasn't it awful and it was painful and this that and the other, and I actually was quite excited by it, really. . . . I was very aware of what was going on, and I found it quite exciting actually, they kept saying 'oh, got an egg' as they kept yanking these eggs out and I was really excited, I mean I was absolutely fascinated by how they were doing it, how they could retrieve these eggs.

As it is undoubtedly the case that a person's attitude can influence the experience of pain, and/or its interpretation, such comments are not surprising, though they were rare. Likewise, retrospective accounts of pain are not only altered through intervening circumstances, but also by the tranquillizers, which can have a mild amnesiac effect.

Far more common than Jennifer Young's excited fascination and enjoyment of aspiration were descriptions of the procedure as very painful and traumatic:

Now the actual experience of having the eggs retrieved, they gave me the valium and the pethadin, and I thought oh this is lovely, this is a lovely feeling, I was sort of floating on air, you know, laying there, and all of a sudden it felt, well, I can imagine as though someone had stabbed me. The pain, oh I just couldn't believe it, and I just lay very still because I remember him saying if you move Mrs Lewis we will lose the eggs, and they will go into your body and that will be it. So of course I had to suffer it and I just lay there and I was sort of moaning sort of thing. When it was done I said to my husband oh it was agony.

(Catharine Lewis)

The operation itself was excruciatingly painful, I mean [the clinician] said he thought I was very unlucky because they actually got eighteen eggs out of me which was a lot more than they thought they would. He said the more eggs they get out of you he reckons the more painful the operation gets, because you know you are not under general anaesthetic, you are just, I was just doped up to the eyeballs with valium and everything and I remember bits of the operation, I remember crying during the operation, I could hear myself crying, and I could hear the nurse saying you are doing very well, it won't be long now, and I could hear [the clinician] saying there's one and there's another one.

(Jane Caldwell)

These descriptions not only convey the pain experienced by several women during aspiration; they also reveal certain features of women's self-image during treatment which are perhaps significant. For example, there is in the latter extract the comment: 'I remember crying during the operation, *I could hear myself crying*', suggesting two different points of view on the self, one from within and one from without, as it were. The shift in point of view denotes the presence of a dual self-consciousness, of a direct self-consciousness ('I remember crying during the operation'), and of a consciousness of self as seen by others ('I remember hearing myself crying'), which is spoken from a point of view analogous to those of the nurses and clinicians, as if Jane Caldwell were outside herself. Lying on the table, looking at her inner abdomen on an ultrasound monitor, which is also being watched by the clinicians as they locate the follicles, it is clear the woman is instantiated in a complex web of mediated gazes, including her own, through which her body is objectified at the same time that her insides are 'disembodied' via the monitor.

This complex process is revealing of the dramatic respatialisation of conceptive events produced in the context of IVF. It is also suggestive in relation to women's position as both subjects and objects of reproductive science.[11]

THE EMOTIONAL DEMANDS OF IVF

Despite the number of women who remarked upon the considerable, and unanticipated, physical demands the programme made of them, nearly all agreed the physical demands were secondary to the emotional and psychological ones. Frances Keating explains:

> I've never in my life experienced anything so much as that, as after I'd been through the programme [and failed]. I thought I'd get on, I'd cope, I'd pick myself up, but I didn't, I didn't, not for a long time. . . . You've gone so far, but you've still come back, and that's the hardest thing. I felt as if I'd gone all the way up to 99 per cent and then I'd had to come all the way back to zero again. And I think that's what it is. You build yourself up, you get yourself so psyched up, I've done it, and then you think, like, I haven't, and I think that's the hardest part. Because I don't think the IVF programme itself is hard.

A similar description is provided by Mavis Norton:

> Because it is, psychologically I think it's a lot worse than physically, and that's even with all the dashing around and the injections in your bottom every morning. . . . Paying for it and doing it is nothing compared with the psychological part of it. . . . It strikes you in your mind . . . because it's easy to get carried away with it.

Mary Chadwick adds:

> Women can take the physical pain. We wouldn't have gone through four attempts of all that pain if we couldn't take the pain. It's the emotional side that's more traumatic than anything. . . . I just literally fell apart through all this treatment because of the emotional side of it. . . . It's difficult to overcome treatment, and I think when couples go in for IVF treatment they have absolutely no idea what they're going in for, or what it actually involves, because going in for IVF treatment you really are on your last resort . . . and also, it's very difficult to explain, but one of the

reasons I did come to the end of it is, as I say, I was so emotionally drained, the physical side I could take, the pain, but the emotional strain that you go through.

As these descriptions make clear, it is impossible ever to forget the importance of the basic, underlying purpose of IVF, which is to have a child. Underlying the demands of the daily IVF regime, the way it 'takes over' as a 'way of life' and the physical demands of the procedure is the continual awareness that the procedure is a woman's 'only hope', her last resort in the attempt to have a child. The impact of this underlying awareness upon all of the other facets of treatment, and its significance in and of itself, cannot be overestimated.[12]

Dealing with failure

Dealing with failure is undoubtedly the most emotionally wrenching feature of IVF. The importance of failure as a component of IVF, again, derives in large part from the way IVF comes to feel like a series of hurdles. This has two consequences. One consequence is that each hurdle represents another point of potential failure, and there are many more hurdles to overcome than are initially appreci-ated, due to the apparent straightforwardness of treatment. Related to this is the consequence that the more hurdles that are successfully overcome, the harder failure is to accept, having 'come so far':

I mean we were told, we were given details of the programme at the hospital, we were told that on day one you take this tablet and day so and so you start taking the injections and then the eggs start developing and day so and so you have more scans, blah, blah, blah, but you may ovulate normally and then you may abandon the cycle. Well, what happened with me was that the drugs that I was taking and the injections and the tablets which was the drug regime at the time didn't or had very little effect so I didn't even produce one egg in the month so obviously they had to abandon it. Now that wasn't something [we'd been told], the assumption I believed was that I would at least produce one egg, although they would expect me to produce anything up to twenty-odd, so that was very disappointing.

(Meg Flowers)

Hence, there is a considerable amount of emotional work involved in coping with the demands of the IVF procedure, particularly when it fails, which is almost always the case. Again, the intensity of the emotional and psychological demands of treatment are often un-anticipated, even when a couple has undergone several cycles and know the routine.

Personal boundaries

Emotional difficulties are also encountered in the context of information management, as it might be described, concerning both fertility problems and their treatment. In response to questions about who they told about IVF, women reported several difficulties related to personal boundaries concerning their treatment. This came up often in relation to paid employment, as discussed below. In addition, decisions had to be made about the pros and cons of telling family and friends, both about infertility and IVF. Some women felt that openness was the best policy, but others felt conscious of continually having to 'keep up a front'. Some women simply lied about their treatment, saying they had to visit the hospital for some other reason. Many found it hard to tell people even if they felt this was the preferred solution. Others found it hard to explain the nature of treatment itself, given the complexity of demands it presented. When telling people about their treatment, some women also found the reactions difficult, thus creating awkward responses to negotiate in addition to the difficulties of disclosure:

> My hardest part was keeping it from the girls at work. And every time I had to go down to [the clinic] during the day I used to tell them I was going to the hospital to be treated for a urine infection. The lies I told, honestly, it's a wonder I didn't have white spots all over my tongue!
>
> (Ruth Levy)

> [Telling people] made it so much worse because there are all the more people to say well it hasn't worked, and there were too many people feeling sorry for me, and I couldn't cope with that either, oh, you know, we are all so sorry, we are so very sorry, and why didn't it happen, what went wrong, and you know, it just went wrong.
>
> (Mavis Norton)

> It's just a difficult topic to sort of talk about, I mean once it's been broached it's not so difficult, because a lot of people have had problems, but just that initial deciding to tell is difficult.
>
> (Sylvia Newton)

> The one thing I got fed up of, I got fed up of talking to people I had to explain the treatment to ... because it can get quite tedious to actually sit there explaining to someone. . . . They don't know the technical part, and you can be sure they don't know the emotional part.
>
> (Jane Caldwell)

Most of the women interviewed found that going through the cycles as part of a group provided the best forum in which to discuss issues related to treatment. As they shared time together in the waiting room of the clinic, which was itself decorated much like many of their sitting rooms at home, the immediate demands of treatment could be discussed with other women at the same or different 'stages'. Although some participants in the study felt that organised support groups, or counselling services, would have been helpful, many had reservations about sharing their feelings among a group of other infertile couples. When asked about support groups, ten of the interviewees said they had reservations even about sharing their feelings among a group of other infertile couples. When asked about support groups, ten of the interviewees said they either had gone to a support group meeting, or would do. Of the remaining, nine said they would not go and in three cases the woman would have gone but her male partner would not.

For three of the women interviewed, organising support groups and acting as informal counsellors to many of the other women on the programme became a major component of their relationship to IVF. In one case, continuing in this capacity after having stopped treatment served as a means of coming to terms with ending treatment. This volunteer work provided by women was thus a contribution over and above the demands of treatment itself, constituting a traditional form of 'women's work', that of nurturing and caring in a volunteer capacity, and by so doing also servicing the clinic by providing a much needed, and freely provided, support service. At the same time, it is also understandable how work of this kind might function as a means of coping with the difficult emotional demands of IVF, including those of serial failure.

REPRODUCTIVE WORK AND PAID WORK

As has been described so far, the IVF routine itself requires a considerable amount of work by the women who undergo it. This work takes a variety of forms, including the work of organising 'the routine', the work of travelling back and forth to the clinic, of monitoring and coordinating the various tasks involved in the treatment cycle, and the physical, emotional and psychological work of coping with the technique's demands. The work of managing information about infertility also occupied the concern of many of the women interviewed, and is usefully described by Sandelowski in her study of US couples undergoing IVF as 'face work' (1993: 81–6). In addition, a number of issues related to paid work were raised during the interviews. Although all of the women interviewed had been involved in paid employment at some point, fifteen out of twenty-two (70 per cent) had either already left or were planning to leave full-time paid employment for reasons directly related to their treatment. It was not only logistical difficulties, but other issues as well which account for the tensions between women's 'productive' (i.e. paid) and reproductive work.

Arranging for cover and time-off were the most significant logistical difficulties encountered by women in the attempt to adjust their paid work with the demands of IVF. Significantly, it was often easier for their male partners to arrange time off work to accompany them to the clinic than it was for the women themselves to do so. Whereas most of the men worked in white-collar, professional jobs, where they had comparatively greater control over their time and their work schedule, most of the women were in jobs which required being continually available in a supervisory or service capacity. A lack of a sense of fulfilment or of future prospects in their paid employment also became apparent in several women's comments about their paid work. While many women expressed a reasonable degree of job satisfaction, many also felt there was little or no opportunity for career advancement, and, by their mid-thirties, most were looking for a change. This ambivalence stemmed in part from the competing demands women felt between their lives as paid workers and the lives they hoped to lead as mothers. As women's lives were likely to be more dramatically transformed by the birth of a child than those of their partners, many had for long periods of time pursued part-time or temporary work in the expectation that they would soon become pregnant, and felt they had essentially put their work futures on hold for a period which had extended much longer than they anticipated:

> IVF only makes life more difficult. . . . I would have had to accept it a long time ago if it weren't for IVF. At twenty-eight I could

have either gone for adoption or accepted my situation so I'd be five years down the line towards that and getting on with my life. Now, you're in a better position to do that when you're twenty-eight than when you're thirty-eight. If you've missed all your career boats, burned all your career bridges because you've spent the last ten years chasing fruitless treatment, you've actually missed out a lot on life.

(Beth Carter)

As Beth Carter, a successful saleswoman, explains, there is not only an evident tension between the demands of productive and reproductive work or identity, but this also introduces an important feature of the IVF experience: how it changes women's views of their life choices over time. This theme is developed further in subsequent chapters. For the purpose of this section, this reflection demonstrates the familiar kinds of difficulties women face in having to choose between motherhood and paid work outside the home, only in this instance it is the attempt to become a mother in the first place which is the source of tension.

Reconciling paid employment with the work of achieving a pregnancy demanded by IVF caused difficulties at both the practical and the emotional level. Logistically, women found it exhausting to maintain full- or even part-time employment during treatment:

I mean it really does take it out of you. I mean I've been getting the earliest appointment possible at [the clinic], nine-o'clock, which means leaving here at half-seven and quarter-to-eight, you dash to [the clinic] because you are in all of that rush-hour, you sit and wait with your bladder bursting, and then you are straight out of there and you are tearing down the motorway again to get back to work. . . . You are breaking your neck, and you feel as if you've done half a day's work by the time you get there, and then before you've even got your coat off it's do this, do that, do that, and you are worn out.

(Mavis Norton)

In the explicit reference to how the demands of IVF come to feel like 'half a day's work' is apparent the appropriateness of considering the demands of IVF in terms of labour. Often invisible as such, like the work of femininity, which, similarly, involves consumption, bodywork, emotional and psychological work, IVF can be described as a form of reproductive labour, or the professionalisation of fertility management.[13]

For some women, paid employment was helpful as a means of coping with the emotional demands of treatment, despite the added burdens it imposed. Meg Flowers found it an essential means of escape:

> Well the job I do, it is an office job but it is very very busy, very very hectic, so luckily most of the day I just don't have time to think about anything to do with me.

Especially as a means of coping with failure after unsuccessful treatment, many women noted the usefulness of paid employment in taking them out of themselves. Catharine Lewis, who had become a nurse after losing a pregnancy very late in term, expressed the following:

> Now they say it either kills you or cures you with nursing – to get yourself stuck into something – and it certainly did the trick. That cured me, and even then I'm feeling depressed but doing the nursing and seeing other people in desperate situations it made me feel well my worries are nothing, that's how I felt.

On the one hand, women's work experiences were an important source of solace and relief. On the other hand, comments such as 'I just don't have time to think of anything to do with me' or 'it made me feel my worries were nothing' are also typical of the ways in which women often neglect their own needs and concerns, or see them as trivial or 'silly'.[14] In addition, such comments reflect the British emphasis upon keeping a 'stiff upper lip' and avoiding disclosure of personal hardship, especially if it is emotionally related.

Paid work provided a fall-back option for many women, who were self-conscious of the risk of 'putting all of their eggs into one basket' (or into a Petri dish) and were careful to protect their work identities. Jane Caldwell, a social worker, was well aware of the dangers of investing too much of herself in the pursuit of achieved conception:

> I was very wary at the beginning, I mean I've come across women who seem to let it [infertility] control their every thought, gesture, life, their whole life is one of failure because they haven't had children and I was very anxious not to end up like that. So I have always, all the way down the line, put a lot of effort into having something else in my life.

> (Jane Caldwell)

Interestingly, Caldwell's comment also indicates the thoughtfulness with which many women decided to undergo IVF. It is important to stress that, at least in this study, women were well aware of the risks they were running by opting for IVF. They were not blindly opting for a wonder cure. Yet also evident here is the kind of 'it's going to work for me' attitude, in the form of not wanting to fail in the ways other women have (see Williams 1988). The wariness described here is a prudent one: it is evidence of having not only seen, but having seriously considered, the dangers of over estimating the likelihood of success.

Despite awareness of its advantages, both in terms of coping with the immediate stresses of IVF, and in terms of preserving future options in case it failed, women often found their paid jobs both exhausting and dispiriting. This was particularly true for women in jobs such as teaching, nursing or social work, where providing cover for absences proved difficult, and was often impossible. Jane Caldwell continues:

> When I left work, which was partly due to the treatment because I knew I was going to have to start going up to the clinic daily, there was no way in my sort of job I could get the cover I needed, because if you are not at work there's only two staff on duty, you can't just pop off to the clinic.

Remaining in full-time, or even part-time work, was also difficult because some women felt their absences were used against them in an exploitative manner. In addition to taking unpaid leave and often less pay, some women felt their employers took advantage of the difficulties their treatment presented:

> We are talking about a firm that is doing extremely well, knows I'm underpaid, uses this [IVF] as an excuse not to give me any more money because they are not sure how long I am going to be there, but I am loathe to leave because I don't know how I will stand benefit-wise if I am out of work for any length of time, and of course if it [IVF] doesn't work, where are you then?
>
> (Mavis Norton)

In this instance, the tension between paid productive labour and reproductive labour was exacerbated by the employer appearing to pit the one set of demands against the other. This is an important reminder of the tensions produced for women in combining paid work and parenting.

Two kinds of work

Going through treatment had, for some women, the effect of concentrating their desire for a family and increasing their dissatisfaction with paid work:

> When I first decided to get pregnant ... I think I was more philosophical about it, just, well, if I get pregnant I do and if I don't I don't. And then the longer it went on, the more I realised I really did want a family, and now I don't know what I am going to do if I can't become pregnant, if I can't have a family, I really don't know how I am going to cope with it. I decided that I'm not really interested in my career anymore. In fact, while I've been off this time we've discussed it and I am going to give up. ... I think it changed my values and my attitudes, it put a different perspective on things, because I've always been conscientious at work and I've always felt it was extremely important, and I'm not saying it isn't important, and I've invested a lot in it, and then when I was pregnant [IVF pregnancy which failed] I realised it wasn't as important to me as I had always thought it was.
>
> (Kate Quigley)

In this statement, as in the opening comment to this section, in which IVF was said to 'only make life more difficult', the experience of treatment has changed the perception of paid work. Here, the initial feeling is described as 'philosophical' towards pregnancy. But with the concentrated attention on getting pregnant involved in IVF, the perception of work changes, 'I realised it wasn't as important to me'.[15]

Dissatisfaction with paid work outside the home, and a sense of its shallowness, of not getting enough back, was also framed in terms of the contrast between waged work in a professional and/or service capacity and the work of being a mother. As Patricia Evans notes:

> My job was always second best to what I really wanted to do, and it got on my wick, and I think it showed in my working capabilities, definitely showed. ... Longing for a little-un really put the kybosh on that job. ... You think what am I doing? Why aren't I pregnant? Why am I still at work? Why aren't I at home looking after a little-un? You know you want to be a mummy and it really gets on your wick that you aren't pregnant.
>
> (Patricia Evans)

The feeling of dissatisfaction with paid employment, and the desire to 'be home looking after a little-un', compounded by the fact that serial attempts at IVF can increase the desire for a child, may also be accompanied by an explicit desire to do the 'job' of being a mother particularly well. It is likely, for example, that women in infertile partnerships will have more fully investigated their desire for children, and given greater thought to what is involved in parenting than many women who have children without these obstacles. Part of the difference between achieved pregnancy and other pregnancies is the amount of careful thought focused around the demands of parenting, and for women especially, the demands of mothering:

> I wish people could see that if every mother did a good job the world would be a twenty-times better place than it is, because that mother is responsible for creating a worthwhile person who is going to live in this world. . . . To do that is such a vital role in life. . . . It's so important and that's why I think part of me drives me on.
>
> (Jane Caldwell)

Here again, the reference to mothers doing 'a good job' underscores the way in which women perceive the work of mothering both as analogous to paid work, and also as of equal, if not greater, importance. Also evident is that they are holding two systems of labour value, the one productive and the other reproductive.[16]

Finally, it is useful to note that in experiencing the conflict between the reproductive work involved in IVF, and their paid jobs, the women interviewed can be seen to be inhabiting merely a different variation of a theme which runs through most women's lives: that of balancing the demands of reproductive work against the demands of their careers. With IVF, the conflict differs in that it is the work of becoming pregnant, of achieving pregnancy, rather than the work resulting from pregnancy, of raising children, maintaining the household and belonging to a kinship network, which poses the conflict.

CONCLUSION

It is because the demands of IVF are so intensive that the procedure comes to feel like a 'way of life', something you 'eat and drink', that you 'live' twenty-four hours a day. This intensity is also produced by the 'obstacle course' nature of the programme itself, involving a constant build-up at each stage, which either leads to another cycle of build-up at the next stage, or leads to the cycle being abandoned, which produces all of the demands of coping with failure. Understanding how IVF becomes a 'way of life' is also important in terms of the wider issues women have to make sense of while they are going through it, concerning their identities, their lives, their relationships and their futures. It is also particularly important in understanding the momentum IVF acquires as a process, and the difference between what it looks like going into it (pre-IVF) when IVF is an option about which a woman may have a lot of information, but by definition no experience, and what it looks like once it has begun, or 'taken over'. Repeatedly, women emphasised that they did not realise how demanding the technique would be, how intensely it would affect them, and how much their lives would feel as though they had been 'taken over' by the technique.

This feature of the IVF experience is also significant because it explains how and why some women change during treatment. As their assessments of the success or failure of the technique itself changed, for example, so too do their assessments of other things, such as how much they want a child, how much they like their job, what a future with or without a child would be like, and so forth. In this sense, IVF is like a rite of passage, through which an individual moves from one state to another. Not all women are changed significantly by experiencing IVF, but all are changed to some degree, and the potential for the technique to shift a woman's perceptions of herself, her needs or her goals is clearly evident in the descriptions of how intense the procedure can be.

This intensity is important to understanding the differences between how women go into IVF, how they then experience IVF itself, and ultimately how they leave it. It is necessary to look at all three of these dimensions of IVF, before, during and after, in order to provide a thorough account of the experience of treatment. Representations of women's experience which focus solely on the way women feel going into treatment therefore exclude much of what is most significant about the experience as a whole. This experience is not static; it is a process, which may turn out to involve considerable and unexpected change. In the next chapter, some of the ways in which the experience of IVF can change women's definitions of wider issues external to treatment are explored, as well as features of IVF as a process over time.

Chapter 4

'It just takes over': IVF as a 'way of life'

INTRODUCTION

In the last chapter, women's experience of IVF was investigated in terms of the most immediate demands posed by an IVF programme, the impact of these on women's lives and the ways in which women 'manage' the procedure. In this chapter, the focus moves to a wider frame, taking into account women's perceptions of their needs, desires and expectations of the technique. It is argued that these are important factors in understanding how women make sense of the experience of IVF not only as a procedure, but as a process over time which involves continual re-evaluation.

In order to understand women's expectations of IVF, then, it is first necessary to consider how these are framed in relation to the experience of infertility. In the first section, the experience of infertility is explored in terms of how it disrupts certain assumptions women held about how they would live their lives, and how they make sense of these disruptions. In other words, this section addresses the ways in which the discovery of infertility contradicts certain features of an assumed worldview, an assumed trajectory of the lifecycle, an assumed sequence of events. In turn, these disjunctures create the opportunity for women to reflect explicitly upon certain needs and desires they feel in relation to parenthood and reproduction and to redefine their reproductive choices accordingly.

It is the way in which women evaluate the disruption posed by infertility, the losses they feel in relation to it, and the options they see before them which will determine their course in relation to expensive, high-tech infertility treatment such as IVF. Cost alone makes this an option available to some women more than others, and some women not at all.[1] But many other factors influence a woman's perception of the IVF option as a means of resolving her reproductive future. The 'logic' of the choice to opt for IVF is not self-evident, and not all women choose it. It is a particular way of evaluating a situation based on a specific set of assumptions and desires which, as is suggested below, lead to IVF coming to be seen as the appropriate and desirable course of action.

Hence, the way in which the disruptions posed by infertility influence the choice of IVF is the subject of section one. It is argued that the choice of IVF belongs to an assumed trajectory of the lifecycle not unlike that depicted in the media representations discussed in Chapter 2. The disruption of this trajectory, and the need for resolution through the attempt to have a child, produce the 'obviousness' of the choice to opt for IVF.

In the second section, a different trajectory is explored; that encountered in the context of 'achieved conception', that is, during the course of IVF treatment itself.[2] Here, a different sequence of events is anticipated, a different set of assumptions about what will occur is established and a different set of 'gaps' open up when, in the majority of cases, treatment does not proceed as hoped. Here, a very different mentality comes into being. In this section, the specific demands of IVF treatment itself are explored, with particular emphasis on the difficult decisions faced by women undergoing treatment and their strategies for negotiating them. This is 'new territory', and there are few precedents to guide women and their partners through the complex demands of treatment.[3] A tremendous amount of determination is required, and is evident, in their accounts of their experiences.

In the conclusion to this chapter, these two trajectories are brought together, in terms of how the one leads on to the other, how they are inhabited and negotiated, and the difficult dilemmas they both produce.

THE DISRUPTIONS POSED BY INFERTILITY

In this section, my aim is not to explore the experience of infertility itself in depth, as the interviews were not oriented to this task.[4] Rather, the experience of infertility is here analysed as *the context out of which the decision to opt for IVF emerges*. Hence, the account offered below of women's descriptions of how infertility affected them are presented with a view to more fully elucidating the ways in which IVF comes to be seen as a desirable 'solution', and the ways that particular hopes and expectations come to accompany the choice of the technique.

Encountering uncertainty

Having taken for granted their abilities to bear children, and, in some cases having already given birth to a child or been pregnant, the discovery of infertility, either their own, their partner's or simply 'unexplained', was for many women difficult to accept, or even to comprehend. This discovery opened up a 'gap' separating them from the life they had expected to lead. It also opened up a number of 'gaps' in relation to their marriages, which they felt could not be 'completed' or 'fulfilled' without a child. Infertility presented an obstacle to the 'normal' and 'natural' progression they had anticipated from marriage to parenthood, and thus from marriage to family. For many women, this had not even been a fully conscious expectation, so self-evident was the assumption that they would have children of their own:

> We wanted children, and I suppose it's like everybody, you just think it's going to happen and you don't think there are going to be any problems and when it doesn't happen it's, you know, it's devastating.
>
> (Christine Ingham)

> And after about three years or so we decided that we would like a family so I stopped contraception and sort of waited to get pregnant, and I didn't. You know you sort of tend to automatically assume that you will, because after so many years of sort of trying to stop becoming pregnant, you sort of think the minute you stop contraception you will become pregnant.
>
> (Kate Quigley)

> Well we started trying for a family . . . and I think I was probably, well I can say it never really occurred to me that I might not be able to have children. I think that's common . . . it's something everyone presumes they can do . . . people do say *if* you get married, they don't always make the assumption that you will be able to get married if you want to . . . so you are always aware of that being an if, but people don't ever sort of talk about *if* you can have children, it's a sort of natural assumption that if you want

them you will have them. Somebody sits there and says I'm going to have two children, I'm going to have one after being married three years and then I'm going to have another one . . . I mean I did that, I'm sure I did that.

(Jane Caldwell)

I think that not to be able to have a family is not something you consciously think about . . . because I think it's a natural assumption to be rather blasé and to think that you assume you are fertile until you are infertile.

(Meg Flowers)

I always wanted to have children. . . . The thought of never having any more was blocked. . . . I couldn't believe I couldn't have children, I couldn't think about that.

(Pauline Harding)

Having children is assumed to be part of a natural and normal lifecycle and the thought that this might not happen had never occurred to many of the interviewees.[5] As the above extracts demonstrate, there are several reasons why the ability to have children is assumed unquestionably. It is described, for example, as an 'automatic' assumption, as 'not something you consciously think about', and as a 'natural assumption'. The ability to bear children is also thought of as a natural capacity, unlike the ability to get married, which depends on social circumstances.[6] Another assumption, which has been noted earlier in the analysis of media accounts, is that of a 'natural' or 'normal' trajectory, in which getting married leads to 'founding a family'. The idea of 'life's progression' through these recognised stages of the life cycle was often cited. As the husband of one of the women interviewed put it succinctly, 'It's the central thing to do, to get married, have children, blah, blah, blah' (Richard Flowers). This trajectory is seen to be both 'normal' and 'natural', and even 'blasé'. It is understood as something 'everyone' presumes:

Well it's something that everyone presumes they – I think it's natural to want your own baby, I think in life you need to reproduce, it felt right, my husband and I get along so well, that was the natural progression, that was the next thing, it just felt right. I mean that's all I can say, it's just nature. I'm a firm believer in nature and what should happen. You should get pregnant and you should give birth and you should follow through with a child afterwards.

(Patricia Evans)

The desire to have children, or to have more than one child, is thus a desire which expresses in part the need to feel that one is progressing along a chosen, expected, or even biologically determined path. The inability to do so therefore creates a disrupted trajectory; expected events are not unfolding as hoped, and a set of expectations of which women were not even necessarily fully conscious beforehand become explicitly recognised in the wake of their failure to conceive as hoped.

Tentative futures

Not being able to have children not only disrupted assumptions about what was normal, natural and right – it also made planning for the future difficult. New plans had to be made, and visions of a future readjusted. The uncertainty surrounding the ability to have children thus creates a tentative future,[7] a future 'on hold' until some kind of resolution is reached. As Liz and Michael Kaplan described it:

> H: So what we decided to do was we had to plan our lives out. If it wasn't going to happen, and it was just going to be the two of us, you know, what, what . . .
> W: What are we going to get from life?
> H: So we both had plans guided out for us so if it does happen great and if it doesn't . . .
> W: If it doesn't, then, you know, what do we do then? What sort of road do we go down? to make our lives as full as possible? Until we knew, you go on for six years, and nothing's happening, you can't plan on anything because you're thinking well . . .
> H: In case it happens.
> W: What happens if I get pregnant next year? the year after?
> H: So you really couldn't get on with the rest of your life because there was always this question . . .
> W: There was always this back of your mind thinking well I may or I may not get pregnant.

Christine Ingham expresses a similar view, again noting the difficulty of planning for the future, and finding it difficult to 'know where you stand':

> But I think it's that, the other reason that makes it so difficult in a way is that you are just left, you don't know what is going to happen, you can't plan for the future, you don't know what you

should do for the best. . . . I think probably that's the most difficult part, you just don't know where you stand, you can't really have a positive outlook on life, because you are hoping for something that just doesn't happen and so it's a very negative situation to be in, isn't it?

Not being able to conceive as had been expected leads to a feeling of not knowing 'which road to go down', or not knowing 'what you should do for the best'. It produces a 'negative' situation in the sense of both an absence and an unhappiness. 'You don't know what is going to happen', because there is always a 'question' in the way of 'getting on with the rest of your life'. From a 'normal' and 'natural' sequence of events, 'life's progression'[8] becomes indeterminate and unpredictable with the discovery of infertility.

For many women, the condition of infertility rendered their futures 'tentative' in so far as they felt unable to fully commit themselves to their jobs or careers as long as the possibility of having children remained unresolved. Many women spoke of 'living in two week spans' or 'living month to month' as they counted the days of their cycles. Of the women interviewed, fifteen (70 per cent) were explicit about the so-called 'treadmill effect' of infertility treatment, whereby a kind of tunnel vision forecloses other options. This awareness was expressed in terms of strategies to ensure a cut-off point to treatment:

I want to get on with the rest of my life, really. I want either to have children or know that I'm not going to have children. I don't want to spend the rest of my life in this limbo. . . . I don't want to just stand in limbo thinking well maybe next year it would work . . . I want to get on with it. . . . Otherwise you are just in this limbo of time ticking on and not knowing, not having any plans for your life at all.

(Jane Caldwell)

'Not having plans for your life' creates a sense of 'limbo' and the sense of not being able to 'get on with it' because of a loss of direction. The feeling expressed here is one of disorientation and frustration, of an aimlessness to the lifecourse. Not being able to have 'plans' creates a sense of being unable to have priorities. Again, the theme of not making progress forward is correlated to an uncertainty about being able to have children.

Feelings of failure

In addition to their futures being rendered 'tentative' and in-determinate, and the lives they had imagined for themselves having been disrupted, many women felt their identities as women were threatened by the inability to have children. This was often expressed in terms of personal failure, inadequacy or guilt. As Beth Carter put it, she was 'not a woman' but more like a 'eunuch' as a result of her infertility. Feelings of failure as a woman, of unnaturalness and of sexual, as well as reproductive, incompetence characterised many women's attitudes to infertility, even when it was not their own: [9]

> I went through stages of different feelings which still continue now but I've come to terms with them better, the feelings of why me, being a failure, and looking at how easy it seems for everyone else to become pregnant is what hits you the most, that sort of feeling of it being so wrapped up in being a woman so you feel it's your failure, your body letting you down somehow. The one time you relied on it to actually do something and it doesn't do it.
>
> (Jane Caldwell)

> As the female I think I was more upset by not having a baby than, I mean, I think really you've got back down to nature, that the whole object of why you're alive really is to reproduce. And if you don't get pregnant, I mean I'd been ready for at least five or six years, and if you're ready, you think 'what am I doing?', 'why aren't I pregnant?'
>
> (Patricia Evans)

> I think you feel inadequate, not quite a woman . . . I still don't feel quite natural. I mean it is difficult to know how it would be, you know, it would be an experience just to be sort of normal.
>
> (Ellen Brown)

> I felt a bit of a failure, I think we both, it hadn't occurred to us that we wouldn't have children . . . so it was very difficult to come to terms with . . . I felt very bitter, why me?
>
> (Jennifer Young)

Feelings of bitterness and disappointment accompany those of failure and inadequacy. Even when the infertility was shared, or likely to be the 'fault' of their partner, some women expressed a feeling that their bodies were 'useless' because they could not reproduce.[10]

I felt my body was useless in that it couldn't even produce a follicle that was going to produce an egg, I did feel, you know, that my body was . . . resentment against my own body. Yes, I did think 'why can't I function normally'?

(Susan Doyle)

The feeling that their bodies had 'let them down' made many women feel unnatural and excluded from normality as well as womanhood. Their bodies thus became an obstacle to fulfilment of their marriages, and thus to the attainment of 'normal' adult status. Pregnancy itself was an experience many women considered necessary to complete their identities as women. As Mary Chadwick describes it:

The whole feeling of actually wanting to be pregnant is very, very strong. Not just because you are going to produce a baby at the end of it, it's just that inner feeling that you have that you need that fulfilment.

Beth Carter described pregnancy as 'wonderful and mystical' and for other women too it was often desired as an experience in itself as much as a child was desired as an outcome. Hence, the inability to conceive left many feelings of inadequacy, both physical and social. The body's incapacity came to be seen as a blockage to a desired trajectory and left feelings of life's progress being on hold while women were left in an unpleasant condition of frustration and uncertainty. In the context of women's frequent sense of inadequacy about their bodies and their sexuality, it is easy to see how the situation of infertility could be interpreted in this way, notably, even when the woman had herself already had children or the problem lay with her partner's body, not her own.

Incomplete marriages

Also important to the expression of desire for 'completion' or 'fulfilment' through having children was the idea of completing the marriage or the family unit:

There's always that little gap that will never be filled. I'd love to be able to be pregnant, to produce a child, to know it's part of us. I'd love to be able to do that, to be able to go through child-birth. . . . It's the only thing I've ever felt I haven't achieved. We've got everything else.

(Frances Keating)

There's something missing, there's something definitely missing
in the marriage.

(Catharine Lewis)

The feeling that 'there is a little gap which will never be filled'
summarises neatly an entire gamut of disruptions posed by the
discovery of infertility. From the most literal level of there being a
mechanical 'gap' in her reproductive physiology (which hence needs
to be 'bridged'), to the 'gaps' in her identity because she is not a full
woman or a mother, to the 'gaps' in her marriage and the 'gaps' in
'life's progression' generally, this is a most apposite phrase to
describe a sense of loss on several fronts. Similarly, the idea of
'completing' a marriage by having children has many components:
raising children together as an extension of the relationship between
husband and wife; having worked hard to achieve a level of financial
security by which to offer children 'a good home';[11] belonging to an
extended family by participating in the activities of childrearing; the
desire to share an activity not defined by the demands of paid,
professional work; and, simply, feeling that having children is part
of the natural and normal progression of married life, some would
say, even its purpose.

The idea of the 'little gap that will never be filled' expresses the
sense in which the gaps opened up by the discovery of infertility are
not only in terms of an expected trajectory, of 'life's progression',
but in terms of relational expectations. The gap referred to here is in
reference to an incomplete conjugality; children are seen to 'complete' a marriage by affirming the relationship between a woman and
her husband, by literally producing a child which embodies a
combination of its parents. This 'completion', like life's continuity,
should flow through a woman's body: it is thus her body which
comes to be seen as the 'blockage' to continuity and completion.

Such an idea is consistent not only with normative conventions,
but with what has been argued to be the symbolic basis of Euro-
American kinship systems, in which the conjugal relationship unites
'the order of nature' (blood ties) with 'the order of law' (marriage).
Children who share an equal genetic ('blood') relation to both
parents both symbolically affirm conjugality and create a dual system
of 'relations': 'blood' relations and 'in-laws' (see Schneider 1968b).
The 'gap' here is thus not only felt in the context of social
expectations, but is arguably a disruption at the level of symbolic
cultural meaning as well.

Although the inability to conceive left many women feeling their marriages were incomplete, or that their marital relationships were 'missing' what a shared relationship to a child 'of their own' would bring, many also spoke of how the quest for parenthood itself, the 'crisis' of infertility, and the experience of IVF, brought them closer to their partners. It was precisely the *achieved* nature of parenthood, or the struggle to achieve hoped-for parenthood, which made it different from what it would have been like if it had happened 'naturally'. In this instance, the attempt to have a child through IVF *itself provided the function desired by the birth of a child*, that is, of bringing the couple together around a shared set of tasks related to parenthood, only, in this case, of would-be parenthood:

> You talk about things much more and talk about your inner feelings, probably more than normal, going through all these things together, it, yes, it has made us closer, hasn't it? It's the seeking after a common goal. . . . I think some people it could drive them apart but with us it has brought us together . . . because it's a shared unhappy time you go through together.
>
> (Sylvia Newton)

Eighty-five per cent of the women who spoke about the effect of IVF treatment on their relationships to their husbands said it brought them closer together. Reasons for this included the effect of being brought closer together by enduring a kind of crisis, or, as described above, 'a shared unhappy time'. Women also felt it enabled men to become more emotionally involved with them, by having to discuss feelings more openly. Almost without exception, though often with a qualifier such as 'men feel things differently', women praised their husbands' supportiveness during treatment.[12] There was also a kind of protectiveness expressed towards men, who were seen as doing very well at something they did not necessarily find very easy:

> He's been very supportive all the way through it. I mean obviously it hasn't been possible for him to come with me every day, you know, and I couldn't expect him to, but he's really been very good.
>
> (Susan Doyle)

Feeling that the treatment brought them closer to their husbands, and affirming their partner's supportiveness, are among the few 'positive' interpretations of the experience of IVF that women expressed. At the same time, some women also expressed a sense of guilt about the burdens they felt their treatment imposed on their husbands:

And in some ways, I, um, (sigh) if I hadn't pursued it and sort of, I mean I wouldn't say I persuaded him because he's not the sort of person who would do anything that he didn't want to do, but I was the one that sort of instigated it and kept it going. And then sometimes I think, well I wish I hadn't done that because now I've brought a lot of hurt and pain to him that he wouldn't otherwise have had, but I mean at the time, I didn't know that would be the outcome.

(Kate Quigley)

I think it's worse in a way for [my husband], because, especially in the first fortnight where there is so much going on, I mean you are thinking, have I done the nasal spray, yes, have I taken the tablets, yes, have I measured me wee, have I taken – I'm busy for at least the first two weeks all the time, now he's got nothing to do. And then there's the waiting, I mean I know it affects him badly, last time when it started to go wrong [he] couldn't cope with it.

(Mavis Norton)

Although it was exceptional for women to be openly critical of their husbands, some did feel the treatment tested their marriages to the point of near dissolution.

Let's just say I can't wait for [this year] to be over, to end, because we've been at it from December to December, and that's it now .... I was just so tired, so uptight that I could feel that what it was doing to us was actually ruining our marriage. ... I didn't want marriage problems, I could see what I was doing to my husband. My excuse was that I was so tired I wasn't interested in sex at all. Then I got to the point where I said I was going to sleep in the other bedroom, I was just turned off completely, I wasn't interested in him at all. I left him and I wasn't going to come back. We really got to that point. But I mean you just can't afford to waste a marriage, having gone through four and a half years of all the trauma that you do go through. ... It's very hard, because you do put your marriage at risk, because of all the emotional strain you go through.

(Mary Chadwick)

Well, basically we have been in infertility treatment for nearly ten years, which is virtually all our marriage and in some ways you, it sort of can spoil the relationship, because it is not quite the same, because it is dominated. . . . It becomes quite focused on schedules, and that side of your life ceases to be private in a way, you feel that, you know, the doctors have sort of probed into it, I mean they have had to, but it does to some extent affect the relationship.

(Ellen Brown)

Like having children, IVF can 'test' a marriage, bringing both positive and negative outcomes. A greater sense of shared closeness, and a sense of pursuing a shared goal can be accompanied by the stresses and strains of coping with the difficulties of infertility and IVF.

Genetic continuity

Yet another important component of the disruption posed by infertility is the desire for genetic continuity through children. What Beth Carter described as the feeling of there being 'no part of me to go on' was expressed by some of the participants in the study. This too was seen as an integral part of completing a marriage, as Susan Doyle explained:

SF: Is it important to you to have a genetic link to your child?
SD: I suppose it is, yes.
SF: What's important about it?
SD: I think it's just something, who can say? It's so very difficult to say *why*, it's just this thing that seems to be in bred in us, isn't it? That you want to somehow carry on through your children and your children's children.

Like the assumption that they would have children, which only became a conscious assumption at the point where its realisation was in question, so too are assumptions about the importance of genetic ties 'just something' so obvious as to not need any explanation.

On the whole, a genetic link was more important to the husband among the couples interviewed.[13] Of sixteen interviews in which the importance of genetic ties was addressed, in three cases it was equally important to both partners, in two cases more important to the woman partner than the male partner, in seven cases more important to the male partner than the female partner, and in four cases equally unimportant to both partners. It is perhaps significant that all but two of the respondents had considered adoption. Three couples had already adopted, of whom two sought infertility treatment to provide a sibling for their adopted child due to the unlikelihood of their being able to adopt a second child. In two cases the husband was not keen to adopt, but in the remaining fifteen cases logistical difficulties, rather than strongly felt preferences, were the main obstacle to adoption. Foremost among these logistical problems was age, while other reasons included one partner having children by a previous marriage, and the long lists and invasive vetting procedures involved in adoption. Hence, for the majority of women interviewed, IVF was chosen over adoption because it was seen as the most expedient means of acquiring a child, not for reasons of preferring a genetically related child.

In sum, the gaps opened up by women's experience of infertility can be seen to be considerable, profoundly affecting several dimensions of their lives. These include the sense of their lives having deviated from an assumed trajectory in which having children played a key role; a sense of their futures being on hold or indeterminate because of this; a sense of failure or inadequacy as women, and in most cases of missing out on the physical experience of pregnancy, which was seen as central to the experience of womanhood; a sense of their lives and their marriages being incomplete without children; a sense that the treatment brought them closer to their partners, but also tested their relationships; and (in a minority of cases) a sense of loss of genetic continuity. The need to resolve these gaps was strongly felt and it is not at all surprising that explanations and resolutions for/of infertility were strongly desired.

There are undoubtedly many women who resolve infertility by simply accepting that 'they were not meant to have children', or that it is 'nature's way' of redirecting their lives in directions they had not expected or wanted but with which they are content.[14] Some women explicitly stated as much, reflecting that they would have accepted their infertility, or indeed had done so, but for the existence of IVF which presented the necessity of re-evaluating their situation.[15] Not all women evaluating the impact of the discovery of infertility would necessarily opt for IVF, and the reasons why the women interviewed did so are explored in the next chapter. However, once they have chosen this route, they move onto a different trajectory, that of IVF itself. In doing so, they are opting for the enablement technological assistance offers as a means of attempting to resolve their situation. It is thus in the hope of finding a resolution that they turn to IVF. Yet, from one 'broken trajectory', in which hoped for events failed to materialise (ie having children, or having enough children, or having a child 'of their own'), they enter another trajectory which presents different hopes and expectations, and different kinds of potential disjunctures. Making sense of this new 'road forward' presents different demands.

THE WORLD OF ACHIEVED CONCEPTION

> I think it would be easier for people if they were told that there was just no way they could have children, then it would be an easier decision to say, well, you know, just tell people that I can't have children and that's it. But most people who do have problems aren't ever told that. You know, they are always told that well this should work, or that treatment should work, you know, it should work this time or we can't find any reason why it isn't happening and or that you've got so much percentage chance of becoming pregnant and really most people aren't told that. I mean the amount of people that go through IVF and only to be told they've had all the tests, but they've been told there's nothing wrong with either of them, you know, so in that situation it's very difficult, it's just a very difficult situation to be in, you know.
>
> (Christine Ingham)

In the effort to resolve the disruptions created by infertility by opting to pursue IVF, women encounter a whole new set of unresolved issues and 'gaps' which need to be 'bridged'. Having come to the technology to *resolve* their infertility, either by producing a child or by being able to say they 'at least tried everything', they in fact often find the procedure opens up whole new gaps and disruptions intrinsic to the trajectory of an IVF cycle. As noted in the previous chapter, IVF is compared to an obstacle course, presenting a sequence of 'hurdles' to overcome. Once immersed in the medical treatment of infertility, particularly IVF, women have entered a very different model of conception. From the 'standard', familiar model of conception in which events unfold along a taken-for-granted, 'natural' and 'normal' trajectory, they enter the model of assisted reproduction, in which conception is not a taken for granted event but has to be achieved.[16] This shift can be seen to be parallelled in terms of ideas about the lifecourse. Instead of having a continuous flow across the 'natural' and 'normal' events of the lifecourse, 'life's progression' is disrupted by infertility, which becomes an obstacle to progress. Overcoming this 'hurdle' is what the choice to undergo IVF is all about. IVF itself is also described as 'like' an obstacle course by many of the women who experience it. Experientially, this obstacle course effect produces a specific set of demands for women undergoing treatment, and it is how the dilemmas produced by the trajectory of treatment itself are made sense of which are discussed below.

Discursively, the field of assisted reproduction is defined by clinical parameters which establish the 'legitimate perspective for the agent of knowledge' and the 'norms for the elaboration of concepts and theories' (Foucault 1976: 199). In other words, what counts as meaningful information in the context of IVF is that which conforms to the established norms and perspectives of the medical experts supervising treatment. For both clinicians and the women they treat, the logic of this definition is obvious: women do not go to clinicians to explore their emotional relationship to their own or their partner's infertility, they go to clinics hoping for a diagnosis, assistance and the desired outcome of a 'take-home baby'.

However, the logic which enables women to accept the terms of infertility treatment does nothing to ameliorate the many dimensions of the experience of infertility and its treatment which are more or less excluded by its established clinical parameters. Having entered into the clinical context of achieved conception, and having accepted its terms, women are left to sort out for themselves the gaps between the medically defined world of achieved conception and the meaning of their reproductive lives outside that frame of reference. The significance of this process becomes clearer in the examples below.

'There is nothing wrong'

A case which illustrates well the kind of paradox this situation can create is that of women who are repeatedly told 'there is nothing wrong':

> You know, the doctor is standing there telling me there is nothing wrong with a smile on his face, and I am thinking, well I actually wish you would find something wrong.
>
> (Catharine Lewis)

> Each test we had they said 'well everything was fine in there Mrs [Levy], everything was fine', and I kept saying I know you're smiling about this, but I wish you would turn around and say you *have* found something wrong.
>
> (Ruth Levy)

In such cases, clinical information ('there is nothing wrong') contradicts personal knowledge ('there is definitely something wrong'). To put this another way, IVF is considered to be a form of 'assistance' to conception. It is represented as 'giving Nature a helping hand'. However, in order to proceed effectively, and in order to 'make sense', the nature of this assistance needs to be specified. Clinically, this problem is simply one of diagnosis. By diagnosing the nature of the infertility, the nature of appropriate assistance is determined. Without a diagnosis, the assistance is more haphazard. Often even with a 'full' diagnosis of the problem, as in the case of blocked tubes, the technique is still unsuccessful. This in turn reveals the partial nature of a diagnosis of the inability to conceive, which is in turn symptomatic of the limitations of any clinical diagnosis, in so far as it depends on partial knowledge from the outset.

Technically, a diagnosis is defined as 'the identification of disease by means of a patient's symptoms' or 'the identification of the cause of a mechanical fault etc.' (*The Concise Oxford Dictionary*, 8th edn., 1990: 321). The problem of 'diagnosing' infertility thus already deviates from the standard definition of a diagnosis in that it is not necessarily a disease, or caused by a disease, and it does not involve one patient, but often involves the interaction between two patients, or more precisely, the gametes of two patients. Perfectly healthy, fertile couples do not always conceive, even when all of the 'required' mechanisms are functional and complete. 'Fertility' is a temporal, and temporary, condition derivative of interaction. Similarly, IVF is not a 'treatment' or a cure, it is merely a bypass operation, 'bridging' a natural deficiency. Women who are infertile are not 'treated' for their physical condition, they are enabled to have a child, or not, despite it.

A problem for both clinicians and scientists in the fields of reproductive medicine and biology, as well as for women and couples who undergo the various forms of assisted reproduction, is thus a gap between information and knowledge. No amount of factual information can compensate for inadequate knowledge, and clinical/scientific knowledge in the context of reproduction is manifestly 'incomplete'. In a sense, there is no such thing as a 'complete' diagnosis of infertility, or, for that matter, of any 'disease'. The point of a diagnosis is instrumental: it is enabling of more effective intervention. One of the problems encountered in the context of achieved conception, both for professionals and for patients, is the problem of making sense of reproduction in a context of evidently 'incomplete' knowledge. This gap between information and knowledge, between the inability to establish a diagnosis and the desire to effect enabling assistance, is precisely the kind of 'new' disjuncture intrinsic to IVF itself.

The parallels between the uncertainty surrounding the causes of conception in the context of IVF, and in debates about conception models historically and cross-culturally, here become especially pointed. As Malinowski's informants were always quick to remind him, heterosexual intercourse does not always produce a pregnancy. For that matter, the meeting of a sperm and egg does not always result in fertilisation, and fertilisation may or may not lead to a pregnancy. Both clinical professionals and couples undergoing IVF know all too well how uncertain the 'facts of life' can be. Despite the vastly increased amount of information available about conception from the procedure of IVF, which extracts the 'moment' of conception from the 'dark continent' of the woman's body (as Freud famously described it), reproductive failure is still poorly understood, and the success rates of assisted conceptive procedures such as IVF have remained disappointingly low. If anything, the increasing amount of scientific and clinical information available about how much can go wrong with the process of conception creates the impression that every baby is a 'miracle baby' (Franklin 1991b).

As noted in the previous chapter, one of the forms of reproductive work involved in IVF is the acquisition of considerable medical expertise about the biogenetic events involved in conception. This takes the form of accumulating a large amount of information which may or may not 'make sense' of the causes of reproductive failure. The following lengthy description of 'being abandoned' for ambiguous reasons expresses well the dilemmas produced by inhabiting a model of achieved conception within which medical information which does not always add up to knowledge, and from which the emotional dimensions of treatment are excluded:

> Well actually, I was abandoned the day before egg collection which was *really* distressing. I found that mortifying, because it was the same again, the follicles were good, there were lots of them, but my oestrogen level had levelled off, which normally happens at ovulation, so there they had left it a day too late, but I'd gone home, had hCG, which is the late night injection which causes you to ovulate, and all through the day they weren't sure, because I had been told yes, everything was fine and you're on

line. Then the consultant had seen the oestrogens and said no, they're not good enough, rerun them, just check them again, if they come back the same she's abandoned, if they come back any better she goes ahead. Now, quite honestly, to be abandoned at that stage is *hell*. Oh, it was just awful. And I had the whole day of waiting to see, and they reran the oestrogens, and at the end of the day they said no, they're no better, that's it. And there is a discrepancy with these figures anyway, so I sort of really hate these oestrogen levels because they've actually been a problem for me all along, and in some ways I wish they would just look at the follicle levels. I don't know, I don't know, it's quite hard for me and what they don't do, sadly, is give you a chance to talk about it.

(Beth Carter)

Here, dependence upon technologically generated information is resented, as its ambiguity causes stress, and its interpretation by the medical staff leads to abandoning the cycle. As Beth Carter describes, inhabiting the medical model of reproduction is threatening in the sense of producing a feeling of being out of control and dependent upon signs and readings which may contain unwanted and distressing outcomes. Also evident is the large and detailed amount of information which does not add up to meaningful knowledge. This information, however accurate and sophisticated, is partial: the oestrogen level necessary for egg extraction to proceed was not attained. No explanation is available, either to the clinician or the patient, for why this is so, therefore throwing future treatment into question, as it is not clear what, if anything, might be done to improve the situation in subsequent cycles.

Decoding the signifiers

Another example of the process of 'making sense' of technologically generated information is the process of interpreting scans. On the one hand, many women found the scanning process reassuring, as it enabled them to 'see' their bodies responding to treatment. On the other hand, because the scanning procedure is one of monitoring reproductive 'performance', and because the activity of her follicles is not under a woman's conscious control, scans could also be distressing, or yield ambiguous 'signs', even to the trained eye:

Well I should say that your second week is – your treatment, things are starting to happen to yourself, in your body. You can't really see anything out of it, for them first few weeks. It's more interesting when you can see your eggs starting to [develop], you see little black patches where they are starting to come, do you know what I mean? It gives you encouragement then, it does me anyway, because I know I can see something coming there, for what I'm having my injections and my treatment and I know that I'm working, starting to work. I know that it doesn't work straight away, but you feel you know, like, even like me, you know. I know I'm at, I know I didn't take completely last time, but I know I have achieved something, I've tried, you know.... I write it down for myself, Sunday I was, I had one thirteen, and I had three size ten, that was on my left side, my right side of my ovary, what had never worked until this time, I've got one a size twelve and one a size ten, that was Sunday. So they both could do well in that time. And then yesterday, one was sixteen, one was thirteen, one was twelve, that was on my left side, so you see they grow a bit each day. They vary day to day, you see, and on my right side the one what was size twelve is fifteen, and that one . . . [end of tape].

(Sara Yates)

I had that element of excitement about it because I was so interested in what was being done. I mean I'd never had a scan before and that was quite exciting, and as I say, I'm interested in the side of how it all works, not just from a will this make me pregnant [point of view], but oh look, that's how the scan works, and I can see the ovaries and so that interested me. So that kept me going really.

(Jane Caldwell)

All I can see is the bladder!

(Pauline Harding)

He'll say 'well there's one' and I'll think well how the heck does he find that? I mean I'd see nothing to do with it, that blotch was nothing. I'd think oh dear, but in the end you got so you could see. But when he used to bring those little crosses down to measure it, I'd think what the hell is he measuring? I couldn't see anything you know . . . It's alright they're saying oh yeah, I can see one or two or three, but I couldn't see it and no matter how my imagination worked I couldn't see them properly.

(Frances Keating)

As these comments demonstrate, the process of making sense out of technologically generated information is represented as both enabling and disorientating. From an initial incomprehension and anxiety ('oh dear'), women come to 'see' their bodies from the perspective of the clinician, a 'way of seeing' through which the follicles become visible and meaningful as signifiers in the context of IVF. The very specific details, such as the sizes of the eggs, are committed to memory, and represent important signs of 'embodied progress'. This is a learned way of seeing: in contrast to the initial impression of 'that blotch was nothing' there is progressive recognition to 'when you can see your eggs'. In turn, this gives encouragement: 'I know that I'm working . . . I know I have achieved something . . . I write it down for myself.' As the last speaker, Frances Keating, describes her second cycle, this transformation becomes evident:

> And the second time 'round, you know, when they brought in the new probe,[17] I, with my left hand ovary, it wasn't always showing up as having anything there and they could never find it because it was always tucked under the uterus, with the normal scan, but using the probe they found it every time, and I could see then, and that made me feel better, I could see that there was plenty there and they were all growing, they were a lovely size. And I think that was smashing, it gave me such a boost. . . . I could see them and I knew then that everything was OK. As soon as they used that probe, yea, I could see them properly, wonderful, and I think that helped.

At one level, then, scanning can be reassuring, indicating that 'everything is OK'. It allows women who have felt their bodies had 'let them down' or 'failed' to see their follicles growing in a manner which has the potential to be interpreted as a sign of, at least, partial 'fertility'. This is a sign of progress: 'So that kept me going really.' The scans can create 'an element of excitement' and of achievement: 'It gave me such a boost.' Yet these signs are always contingent – in Frances Keating's case everything was not 'OK' and the cycle failed. As Rayna Rapp has argued in her ethnographic work on prenatal screening, technological assistance to reproduction involves complex relationships to technologically-generated information which does not always add up to meaningful or useful knowledge (1996). The complex renderings of the 'facts of life' do not always 'make sense'. This hermeneutics of achieved conception, both intimate and at the same time 'objective', creates particular demands which must be continually negotiated. These include developing a 'way of seeing' the scans. Their visual interpretation is a learned, acquired skill, transforming an experience of seeing 'nothing' to one where 'you got so you could see'.[18]

Clearly, the most difficult situation is where the 'signs' do not add up to any meaningful interpretation, in other words, where the cause of the infertility is 'unexplained'. It is generally assumed as a rule of thumb in approximating the causes of infertility that a third of all cases are caused by the female partner, a third by the male partner and a third by a combination of the two partners. Among the couples represented in the sample, the causes of infertility were largely unexplained. Only five cases, in which the women had blocked tubes, and two cases of diagnosed male infertility yielded 'identification of a mechanical fault' sufficient to account for infertility. In the remaining (majority) of cases, the infertility was either wholly unexplained or only partially so, where 'faults' were identifiable, but insufficient in themselves to explain the infertility.

The problem of making sense of conceptive failure was thus, for many women, a major source of frustration. Jeanette Ives describes this 'not knowing all of the time' as follows:

> When they said [IVF] was the only way I could have [children], I came to that decision because, like you do, we just assumed that you have the operation and things are going to be fine. And when they said everything was fine [e.g. the tests] . . . same with the first IVF treatment, great, the eggs were lovely, everything is fine, you know, we can't find anything wrong, and then you'd ring up two days later and they'd say sorry, it didn't work, and we'd say, well why, you know, if everything is fine? I think I'd accept it more if there was, if they'd said the egg count is not high, or the sperm count is not high. Then you would know, and you would know what they are treating. It's this not knowing all the time.

That 'not knowing all the time' causes such frustration is not only the result of lack of knowledge. It is also the result of *the promise of knowledge which has gone unfulfilled*. It is the promise of enabling knowledge and effective technological intervention represented by IVF which leads women to see it as a 'chance', a source of 'hope' and hence as an 'opportunity'. The entire field of reproductive medicine and biology is instrumental in this sense: the promise of knowledge is the control it offers over the reproductive process.

Unexplained failure

That 'everything is fine' in the context of no apparent 'faults', while perhaps initially reassuring and intended to be so, has the potential only to add to the frustration of failure, when it becomes apparent that everything is not fine. It is for this reason many women wanted 'something to be wrong', despite this appearing paradoxical. Kate Quigley explains why IVF can make a difficult situation even harder:

> You know, in some ways it would have been easier if they had said well you've got this problem and there is nothing we can do about it, you never will become pregnant, in a way it might have been easier to accept. But it's quite frustrating for them to say well we can't find anything, you think there must be something, and you think well what is it? And I got pregnant before, so what's different now? And I just sort of keep thinking, you know, why could I then and why can't I now, and, you know, what's wrong? It's the same with IVF in some ways. It might have been easier if it had never worked. But because it started each time, and yet each time it doesn't carry on I might have accepted it and thought, well, I've had a couple of tries and it's obviously not going to work, and yet I think well there's a chance.

For Kate Quigley, two 'successful' IVF pregnancies had ended in miscarriage. Such a situation is especially difficult for obvious and also significant reasons. For one, 'failure' is harder the more 'successful' the procedure has been. Also, a stark contrast emerges between evident 'fertility' and continuing childlessness. Hence the feeling that 'it might have been easier if it had never worked', which could be taken to refer both to the technique of IVF and the woman's own fertility.[19] Most frustrating of all is the knowledge that 'there must be something wrong' while it is impossible to 'find anything'. This leads to the feeling that 'it might have been easier if it had never worked', which is immediately contradicted by the feeling of 'and yet I think well there's a chance' – which sequence neatly encapsulates the ongoing rationale supporting the choice of IVF.

Not surprisingly, failure is easier to accept when there is at least 'a concrete reason':

> They kept saying there's no reason why you shouldn't become pregnant. . . . And I wished they could have given me a concrete reason. I think if they'd said there is no way you could have children, I could have accepted it, but it is all this well you know

we can try this and it might happen and there's no reason why it shouldn't.

(Jennifer Young)

It seemed to be very much trial and error, because nobody ever found anything wrong with either of us, so we didn't feel as if, I've to think what I'm trying to say here, but I never felt as if anybody ever found out what was wrong.

(Sylvia Newton)

The difficulties of coping with unexplained failure in the context of an individual cycle are closely related to the problems of coping with much larger questions such as how long to continue treatment. Even when a 'concrete' reason is found, it is not an explanation so much as a description. Hence, a woman may fail because her oestrogen levels were too low, which might be seen as related to the drug regime. But this is a very partial explanation; it is in fact only a mechanical description. In such circumstances, some women express the desire to be rescued from limbo, even if by the 'worst' news, which would at least provide an end to the stress of uncertainty:

There's just a part of me that thinks why hasn't it worked for me so many times? Shouldn't I have got pregnant after all those goes? . . . Nobody has ever said to me 'the reason you haven't got pregnant is . . .'. What they've *always* said to me, without fail, is 'I really don't know why you haven't gotten pregnant, but I thought you would do, and I'm sure you will'. Now that's terribly nice, but when a few times I've said I don't think I'll go through it any more, it's too much, 'Oh but you will be successful, you must go through it some more'. That's not a fair burden. In some ways, if they'd said to me, you're never going to get pregnant, I'm sorry, this is it, I could cope with that. I can't cope with the idea that, you know, there's just some minor adjustment to be made.

(Beth Carter)

As Beth Carter notes, the search for a resolution in the context of IVF is hampered by the lack of explanation for the high percentage of failures.[20] As several of the comments suggest, this feature of treatment can be so distressing as to lead women to wish they had never undertaken treatment to begin with. It is in such a context that appreciation of the reasons that lead women to choose IVF is useful to understanding the experience of the IVF procedure. Seen from this perspective, it is possible to appreciate the extent to which IVF is difficult *because it exacerbates the very situation it was undertaken to relieve*. In the same ways that women can feel their lives are 'in limbo' as a result of infertility, so they can feel their treatment is 'in limbo' because of the lack of a diagnosis. One set of distressing circumstances caused by an unexplained failure (infertility – 'why me?'), is simply replaced by another situation of unexplained failure ('Shouldn't I have gotten pregnant?'). One version of unresolved futures has led to a different version of the same problem.

The similarity of these situations is also evident in the responses to them. The response to infertility was to do something about it. Likewise, in the context of unexplained infertility, greater determination is required to maintain faith in the enabling potential of IVF despite not having an accurate understanding of exactly what kind of intervention will be successful.[21] *It is in this context that the quest for a child through IVF can become an end in itself.* As each failure yields some diagnostic clarity on the situation, it increases the possibilities for the next treatment to be more successful. Or, having succeeded in reaching a certain stage of treatment in one cycle, the hope of proceeding further in the next cycle is increased. This matrix of determination, failure and hope for success is a definitive feature of the IVF experience, and is discussed in more detail below.

Coping with failure

Coping with failure is undeniably the most emotionally demanding aspect of IVF. While the physical demands may be taxing, many women felt the emotional demands were far worse. While infertility is often described as akin to the grief and sense of loss accompanying bereavement, the problem of infertility in the context of IVF is that it becomes a *tentative condition*. There is a seriality to the experience of grief and loss which would not characterise a bereavement, which is final and by definition singular.

In describing the emotional work involved in undergoing IVF, many women emphasised the importance of balancing hope for success against awareness of the likelihood of failure. Hope for success and preparedness for failure are the opposing extremes of the IVF mentality which must be held together, and somehow balanced. This 'balance' between opposing potentialities was always difficult, and often unsuccessful. Too much hope was seen to lead to devastating disappointment. Too much preparedness for failure was seen as potentially damaging to the outcome, as in a self-fulfilling prophecy, or by creating a level of discouragement incompatible with continued treatment. Meg and Richard Flowers described this as a 'grey area' of ambiguity:

MF: There is very much a feeling that you get from the medical staff that you've got to be realistic about the programme, which I think means that you are not to, I don't know what it means actually, it appears to mean . . ..

RF: On the one hand they want you to be positive about it and on the other hand they want you to be prepared to fail. But they don't really understand the emotions that are involved.

MF: It's very difficult to . . . that sounds very black and white, and it's something that can easily be said by someone who is not participating, but there are so many shades of grey in between. It's like saying be realistic, so expect the possibility of not succeeding, either in this attempt or ever, but you've got to be positive enough to be going through – you've got to want to succeed, but if you don't succeed you've got to accept it. Now to me, that's well, not just thinking about it, but in actuality, that is a very difficult psychological thing to come to terms with. . . . It's a really difficult thing to try and find an equilibrium.

These 'shades of grey' (also discussed by Sandelowski 1993) represent the most obvious liminal component of IVF as a rite of passage. As Victor Turner and others have noted, all rites of transformation run the risk of failure, which is why liminal social beings are marked off from society. Part of the stigma of IVF perceived by many women and couples in this study no doubt derives from the sense of liminality and precariousness the technique involves. As a classically modern liminal space, the IVF clinic reduces women and couples to their biological selves, and strips them of their external identities, while they endure physical, psychological and emotional alterations as part of a quest for clinical transformation.[22]

Other women interviewed also described the difficult balancing act required to cope with failure.

And then each time, you know, they give you some treatment, then you start sort of hoping again, you know, and then it doesn't work, so um, you know, you begin to think it will never work and then you try something else, and it just goes on like that in a cycle until you just accept it in the end that that's it, you know.

(Christine Ingham)

[You can't] raise your hopes at all ... you've got to be sort of half and half. Raise your hopes a little but don't get too disappointed and it's a good thing. It's a good thing to just go in for it, not too pessimistically, but not too oh well what's the point, you know, but not too euphoric and too oh it's definitely going to work.

(Catharine Lewis)

And all this time you've got so many emotions going on in your head, that you daren't get happy anyway. I suppose I'm a bit resigned to the fact that I probably won't ever have any. That's the only way to be.

(Mavis Norton)

I mean I know they say to you they don't guarantee success. They tell you that. But you still say I might be one of them one per cent. And I think every woman that sits in that chair will think the same thing. You think well I'm going to be one of those one per cent. . . . Well they say you've got to go there thinking, well, alright, alright, I might not be successful. But in your heart of hearts you *don't* go in with that attitude. I mean you sit down and talk to them and they say 'you do realise there are no guarantees' and, oh yeah, we know all that, but you don't, not really, inwardly you're saying 'I'm going to do it', you think so positive, and I think that's what it is.

(Frances Keating)

Failure in the context of IVF is never absolute. Both failure and success are continually subject to redefinition, both during and after treatment. Some cycles are considered not to have 'failed' because they did not proceed far enough, and are thus not even considered 'real' attempts. Frances Keating describes one such failed attempt on her first cycle:

On the first cycle they did a retrieval but they only got one good egg, as they thought, but then it fertilised, but it wasn't good enough to put back, so I didn't even get as far as the embryo transfer the first time, which was soul-destroying, because you go through all those up to your seventeenth day for the egg removal to get there and to actually be lying on the table and you know before you've even come off that it's a failure. And I think that was the worst, you haven't even got off the starting blocks, that's how I felt.

In other cases, failure is defined as a 'success' relative to previous failed cycles which fell at earlier 'hurdles'. Hence, even if a treatment fails it is sometimes considered a success in relative terms. Another means by which a failed cycle can be redefined as a successful one is if it yields any diagnostic evidence of potential benefit to future treatment cycles. In both of these cases, 'failure' becomes an impetus to proceed, subsequent cycles being undertaken with a greater degree of hope for success. It is by this means that a failed cycle can be resolved or coped with by undertaking subsequent cycles. This is part of the so-called 'treadmill effect' of infertility treatment, a cycle of dependency on subsequent treatments to resolve failed ones and an increasing determination to succeed in the face of serial failures:

> And then when it didn't work, as I say, I felt pretty awful, but only for a few days, then I started to pick up and think, well next month another attempt, you know.
>
> (Jane Caldwell)

> I don't know whether we would have tried again had they not pointed out that progesterone problem and said that we could do something about it. [. . .] If they had said, well we honestly don't know why it didn't work, it should have done, then, you know, what's to say that exactly the same thing is not going to happen again next time?
>
> (Mavis Norton)

While failure at one of the later stages of treatment can be redefined as a relative 'success' in retrospect, such failures may also be the most difficult to cope with, 'having come so far' only to have their hopes dashed. Descriptions of the aftermath of dashed hopes were incorporated into the cyclical temporality of IVF, in terms of a build-up of expectation, followed by devastation, in turn followed by renewed determination:

> And then even months afterwards I'd be sitting here doing something, I'd be having a cup of coffee, while I was doing something I was fine, but the minute I'd sit down I'd start crying, you know, [my husband] would phone because he does many times during the day, and he would say what the earth's the matter, and I would say I don't know, I just don't know. My character had completely altered, really, I was always a confident person, I knew what I wanted, and I got on and did it, nothing used to bring me

to tears like that. Not just to sit down and cry. I mean if somebody walked through the door, especially my Mum, if my Mum walked through the door, oh, out it would come, I'd just start crying. I found that very hard. It's only in the last month that I've gotten myself together. [. . .] I've never in my life experienced anything so much as that, as after I'd been through the programme. I thought I'd get on, I thought I'd cope, I'd pick myself up, but I didn't, I didn't, not for a long time. [. . .] You sort of have to come back. You've gone forward so far, but you've still come back, and that's the hardest thing. I felt as if I'd gone all the way up to 99 per cent and then I'd had to come all the way back to zero again. You build yourself up, you get yourself so psyched up, and I think that's the hardest part.

(Frances Keating)

It is because of the difficulties of coping with failure, and the necessity of 'hope management', that is, of balancing a sufficient measure of hope against a realistic appraisal of the likelihood of failure, that a certain kind of psychological determination is required to continue with IVF. In meeting the psychological demands of IVF, women and their partners were frequently explicit about conscious strategies they had developed in order to cope effectively. Sylvia and Bob Newton tried a range of strategies to cope with the procedure:

BN: One of the things which we did . . . was to concentrate our minds on eating healthily, to take an interest in what we were eating.

SN: Well I'd seen my friend going through treatment and getting stressed, so when we started . . . we started eating better, etc., and I thought well I'm not going to get like that, I'm going to sort of take it easy and take what comes, hopefully, you know, I will get pregnant without all these problems, but it just didn't work like that. No, I mean I felt stressed a lot of the time which made me very irritable at work, the pressures of going through this and going to work, and we did read up about it, but to actually try to sort of eliminate stress is very difficult. I mean we go to yoga and things like that. We also joined a badminton class as well because I wanted to feel I was doing things other than work. I am a teacher which involves a lot of work at home and I wanted to get out for two evenings a week and do something more relaxing. And people have said to us, oh, well it worked for you because you felt so much more positive about it, and weren't under all the stress that you were before, so I mean it could be true, I don't know.

Other women turned to alternative healing practices to enhance their chances of success and cope with the stresses of the procedure. Beth Carter felt hypnotherapy had significantly improved her mental attitude:

> I went through hypnotherapy before [the cycle I'm on now] and it's extraordinary how much it has helped. I've actually gone through this whole procedure believing it will work, and enjoying it, enjoying it far, far more and finding it less stressful ... I feel as though I'm pregnant now, I imagine that I am, there's no way I could feel it if I really was, but I've gone through it thinking this is going to work and this is positive, and it's been a lot better. . . . Always before I've never thought it was going to work, and I've never allowed that to even enter my thinking, and if I did, just imagine, what it was like, I would be in tears very quickly and it would be very difficult to cope with. . . . I remember on a few occasions thinking how I will feel if they tell me I'm pregnant, and it was so overwhelmingly wonderful, oh it was just lovely, and very moving, and then I'd find myself just in tears thinking of how it would feel, I still could if I, no, I wouldn't, I feel differently now, and I, then I'd push it down again and I actually feel that I never thought it would work, and I wonder, you know, if you don't believe something's going to work if it ever will?

The work of 'hope management' is complemented by strategies such as 'thinking positively' and trying to implement measures to improve the quality of life. In these statements are apparent the explicit, conscious strategies, often the acquisition of a particular mental attitude, which are seen as necessary to continue the pursuit of an elusive goal. This is a major component of 'living IVF' psychologically; it requires deliberate internalisation of a particular mentality. Re-imaging and re-imagining the body itself was another strategy described to enhance chances of successful conception. In an intriguing elaboration on the 'way of seeing' the insides of the body induced by scanning, Meg Flowers describes how she imagined her endometriosis 'exploding' and 'disappearing' in order to think more positively:

> [After failing the first time] I knew I'd got to be a lot more prepared for it, so as for preparing myself psychologically [I did] lots of positive things. After the operations, I'd had the doctor who did

them, each time I see him he sort of says, you are a terrible mess you know inside. Well that might well be a fact, but I don't want to know that, that's a negative thing. I know that there are things wrong with me, but I've got to concentrate on the positive things, because, for example, I know I've got nothing wrong with my womb, and to me that is one of the most important things, I know I can carry a baby if I'm pregnant, so that's a very, very important thing, so now I also think instead of worrying about this endometriosis, because it isn't something that just goes away, if you are not doing anything to stop ovulation then it can come every month and you can get worse every month, it's like a Catch-22, the only way to stop it is to stop the ovulatory cycle, which is, yeah, to me Catch-22 if you want to have a family. So I've now decided I don't want endometriosis, not that I've got it or I might get it, but that I don't want it, and I'm not going to have it, so, it probably sounds a bit daft really I suppose, but if ever I think I might have it, or I have a painful period and I think of I might have it again, I imagine it in my mind and I imagine these little spots of endometriosis exploding, disappearing, so you know I'm not having it because it's interfering with what I want so I'm not having it, and [the doctor] telling me things about oh there's scar tissue here and there and everywhere, so I consciously imagine my ovaries. I've got bits and pieces sewed together, so I imagine them as being perfect, and I imagine the Fallopian tubes as being wide open and perfect, so in my mind's eye, although this doctor keeps telling me it's a dreadful mess, I'm not believing that, I don't want to listen to that . . . I like to think that what I'm feeling is having a positive effect on my body because I wanted it to work, and I know I can do it in the end, it's just sort of having these stumbling blocks in the way, so those are a few, ah, daft things that might help [laughs], well, they help me, I feel a lot better thinking so much more positively about them.

In this description, quoted at length because of its detailed rendering of a particular mental coping strategy, there is an interesting resistance to the medical model of 'mechanical faults' in favour of a more 'positive image'.[23] Such a strategy not only indicates the kind of mental strategising considered necessary to 'self-management'[24] in the context of IVF, but also suggests a dual self-consciousness whereby a woman both inhabits and 're-visions' a medical definition of her reproductive capacity. Hence, whilst the medical definition of her ovaries and Fallopian tubes is accepted at one level (in that she is undergoing IVF), it is also rejected at another (as causing her to feel too 'negative'). Most importantly, this extract demonstrates precisely how IVF is 'lived' in terms of personal identity, by adopting complex strategies of psychological prepared-ness. A particular version of self-fashioning specific to the context of IVF can be seen in this description, based on a re-imagining of reproductive potential in the service of 'positive thinking'.

THE IVF COMMITMENT

Meg Flowers's account is also suggestive of the tremendous amount of determination required to undergo IVF, since the odds are against women succeeding at the outset, and the technique itself is very demanding. Again the obstacle course analogy is appropriate to describe the situation, suggesting as it does the need to acquire the corresponding mindset required of a competitor. These extracts also demonstrate the very particular kinds of psychological demands intrinsic to the experience of IVF, and the ways in which 'making sense' of the experience can be quite demanding, requiring determined strategies of mental self-preparedness to negotiate a 'path forward'.

This determination can bring its own rewards. As already noted, some women felt the experience of treatment brought them closer to their husbands through the shared 'ordeal' of struggling to succeed against the odds. Some women also felt a sense of teamwork, of being at the centre of a medical quest for success, where their hopes were shared by dedicated professionals.[25] This feeling was reinforced by comparisons to bad experiences of NHS treatment where they had felt, at best, neglected, if not grossly mishandled:[26]

> Yes [the clinic staff] are wonderful. . . . And it's marvellous, it is just a nice and relaxed atmosphere, you talk to them on first name terms, and there is no shouting like they do at the women's hospital.
>
> (Stephanie Quinn)

> At least you can look back when you are in your early forties or whatever and say well I did try, I had three good tries, four good tries, OK, it didn't work, but I did try, and at least you know you've had a go. And there's all those people working really hard at the clinic, they all want to make you pregnant, they are all battling, the embryologist, the doctor, all of them, as a team. You know,

they are battling to help you. You owe it to them as well, because without them, what would we do?

(Cindy Cooper)

In the language of a 'battle' for pregnancy, Cindy Cooper clearly indicates the epic genre of self-representation which often characterises IVF descriptions. The 'soldier' mentality, of going to war against the odds, backed up by state of the art technology, interestingly regenders conception narratives. Far from the 'lie back and think of England' narrative of passive acquiesence to nature in the service of the nation, IVF pronatalism is narrated as an aggressive pursuit of an elusive goal, in which women are warriors, with battle scars attesting to their bravery on an epic quest for a child of their own. Passivity is not a virtue in the world of achieved conception.

The achieved nature of pregnancy in the context of IVF is also apparent in the emphasis on a team of committed professionals who 'all want to make you pregnant'.[27] Only two of all the interviewees failed to praise the clinic staff, often in glowing terms. The opportunity to feel they were being taken seriously and kept well informed, as well as feeling reassured that everything possible would be done for them, was frequently noted. Very much in contrast to ethnographic accounts of high-technology birth (Davis-Floyd 1992), in which women often feel at odds with the medical personnel commanding their bodies to behave like machines, women undergoing IVF at times express almost euphoric appreciations of the clinicians they see as their comrades in struggle. Significantly, this contrast was often embedded in the contrast between the impersonal and often rude behaviour of the NHS staff versus the customer-satisfaction orientated service of private healthcare professionals.

They couldn't have been better. They explained everything . . . [they said] come and talk to us if you want to change the drugs or the treatment or whatever. They were very nice. As I say, they explained all of the possibilities that they know of. Very helpful.

(Jeanette Ives)

They were brilliant, really, you can't fault it, I mean they were so caring with you. . . . I mean on most of the NHS it seems to be like a cattle market.

(Frances Keating)

They've been fantastic, absolutely fantastic . . . I'm not just saying this because I'm preganant . . . I mean really, what they do there is absolutely fantastic. They're just miracle creators, absolutely fantastic! [pause] And they're so patient and so gentle, the staff, the crew they've got there . . . they're only eager to help you.

(Ruth Levy)

Being at the centre of a team effort, aided by a 'fantastic crew' of 'miracle creators', who are 'brilliant', 'caring' and 'helpful', as well as professionally dedicated, could not be further from most women's previous experiences of reproductive healthcare, many of which had been appalling, and even life-threatening, due to negligence. As noted in Chapter 2, these comments also reference the emergent 'two-tier' health system in Britain, whereby those who could afford to pay for private health services had access to superior care. Compared to 'the cattle-market' of 'the women's hospital' and 'the NHS', a strong contrast is apparent in the 'patient' and 'gentle' staff who are 'eager to help'.[28]

The radicalism of the Thatcherite redefinition of a sense of national belonging is also evident in these contrasts, through which the ability to reproduce is evaluated in terms of the enterprise culture analogy. In contrast to the traditional relegation of procreative acts to the domain of the personal, private and domestic sphere, the emergent consumer culture of conception services clearly demonstrates the embeddedness of wider political and economic changes at the very heart of conjugal intimacy. Reproductive freedom in this context is redefined as consumer choice and customer satisfaction. In relation to citizenship, the right to purchase services, such as private assisted conception options, interestingly recombines nationalism, pronatalism, familialism and the value placed on a free market economy.

The ironies of women's appreciations of improved healthcare under Thatcherism (which, on the whole, depleted many public women's healthcare programmes and particularly adversely affected women healthcare workers[29]), many women I spoke with for this study clearly felt empowered by their experiences of private infertility treatment. Not surprisingly, the combination of a sense of teamwork, achievement and determination to succeed often made women comment that IVF had 'made something of them'.[30] Not unlike an Outward Bound course, of sorts, it had given them a sense of hard won accomplishment:

As I said, I've always been a very determined person, if I want something I go out and get it. . . . I'm stronger willed I suppose

than I thought I was. Everybody says I'm easy, and too soft, and
I suppose people didn't think I would be able to go through all this
[but] I was quite certain in my mind that this was it, I was going
to try everything, no matter how much it cost or how much it
pained. . . . It brought out a strength of character I didn't think I'd
got, you know, because you've got to be strong enough to cope
with it.

(Jeanette Ives)

It's a funny thing really, it's a hard programme but it really makes
something of you.

(Frances Keating)

I think the whole traumatic experience, although it's awful, I
think it does make you accept that you can't have everything in
life and things aren't just given to you on a plate. You know, some
things you've got to work for, and I mean it sounds ridiculous, but
we've had to work for it, you know, eventually, and it's taken us
six years.

(Susan Doyle)

Having to *achieve* pregnancy, even though it is 'traumatic', is
appreciated for being a greater accomplishment than having children
would have been 'normally'.[31] Whereas most couples 'take for
granted' their ability to reproduce, women who undergo IVF can
feel, as the last speaker states, that achieved parenthood is special
because it is different: a unique accomplishment. In this too lies an
important component of the meaning of 'achieved' conception. It is
different, it 'makes something of you', and it is all the more valued
as a result.

It was this determination which led women to choose IVF, *even
when they thought it was likely to fail*. The determination to do
everything possible, and even to test themselves in the process, was
very strong. This determination can become an end in itself, ironically coming to serve many of the functions that having a child was
expected to provide, such as proving oneself, providing a focus for
the marriage, dedicating shared resources to the quest for parenthood, and so forth.[32] It is in the conjuncture of women's determination
to do everything possible to attempt to achieve a pregnancy, and the
clinician's offer of enabling technologies of reproductive assistance,
that an 'obvious' trajectory out of the 'hopelessness' of infertility
comes into being. Once on this trajectory, determination to succeed

against the odds, while facing the challenges of IVF, becomes a potentially rewarding activity in itself, despite the high costs.[33]

At the time of their interviews, all of the women I spoke with said they would recommend IVF. Without exception, they praised the technique, and many considered themselves fortunate or 'lucky' to have been able to undergo treatment. By so doing, they were also affirming their own decision to have opted for IVF as a means to resolve the disruptions posed by infertility. Of course, such affirmations of the technique and of their own decisions are hardly surprising, especially in a context where hope for success was considered critical to its realisation. Doubtless, some women would later have regrets, or indeed at the time had reservations they did not express, possibly even to themselves.[34]

CONCLUSION

While this determination and positive assessment of the technique cannot be considered representative, it does indicate how much variation and contradiction is part of the experience of undergoing IVF. Despite its costs and pains, it is not only possible for women to endorse the technique, but even to feel it has 'made something of them' as women. In order to appreciate the reasons why women opt for IVF, a technique with an overwhelming rate of failure, acute demands, high costs and taxing emotional and pyschological, as well as physical, requirements, these ways of 'making sense' of treatment must be appreciated. They demonstrate how IVF as 'a whole way of life' rests on the promise of enablement through technological assistance, and the maintenace of hope against the odds that it will succeed. It is defined by a sequence of obstacles that pose a constant challenge to women who undergo it which they meet to the best of their ability, using a range of strategies to cope, and demonstrating a sophisticated self-awareness in the process. Their observations of how the technique affects them, in terms of their sense of self, their relationships, their work and their futures were often remarkably frank, honest and perceptive. As a 'way of life', IVF was something they coped with ably and knowledgeably, an appreciation that must be borne alongside the very justifiable concerns about IVF as a means of alleviating infertility.[35]

From the perspective of anthropological theories of kinship, IVF raises a number of important questions. The Schneiderian view of kinship as a cultural system, for example, foregrounds the central importance of heterosexual intercourse as a means of establishing conjugality and procreativity. This, he argues, is because of the capacity for the 'natural facts' of reproduction to operate as a legitimating and sustaining symbol of the essence of kinship and marriage. Yet, in the context of achieved conception, the instability of this 'dominant' cultural logic is exposed: the pursuit of conception through highly artificial means *can function equally well as a unifying goal*. At once commensurate with the underlying logic of kinship, parenting and marriage, and also disruptive of this logic to a very great extent by 'denaturalising' it, the pursuit of achieved conception raises important questions about the relationship of procreative desire to principles of social organisation. As Strathern has argued, assistance to conception unsettles the naturalising function of procreative unity in the form of a child who is the shared progeny of both parents (1992b). Implicit in the choice to opt for IVF is the introduction of technology as an enabling force in the production of new persons. This third party to the procreative conjugal unit has an effect of displacement: the authorising principle of natural facts as the irreducible essence of heterosexual family formation is 'assisted'. In turn, this 'assistance' troubles the capacity for nature to authorise conjugal unity. In place of 'nature', conjugality becomes defined by choice, consumer choice, as enterprising citizens avail themselves of technoscientific options to achieve personal fulfilment. Yet, unlike 'nature', whose trajectories are by definition beyond the scope of full human mastery, consumer choice and technological enablement represent new freedoms to construct the future, be it individual, national or global, according to precise specifications.

IVF as a technique poses particular demands, as is well evidenced by this study. Yet these demands are in other respects not particular to IVF. Condensed in the IVF story, as it is narrated by those most closely connected to it, are wider stories about how the future can be imagined and pursued. In the conjuncture between reproduction and technology are combined two of the most powerful Euro-American symbols of future possibility: children and scientific progress. It is for this reason that the IVF story is inevitably concerned with the meaning of progress, the character of hope, the desire for children and the will to overcome adversity. In these stories too are evident the particular constellations of management, instrumentalism, self-fashioning, and consumerism specific to a particular time and place. To the extent that anthropology seeks to locate its own endeavours at cultural explication more fully, it must put into dialogue the long history of its models of kinship, conception, procreation and personhood with the singular refrain on these concerns provided by contemporary Euro-American redefinitions of 'the facts of life', the givenness of ideas of the 'natural', the incursions of consumer choice into the production of new personas, and the role of technology in 'troubling' many other taken-for-granteds about the human condition.

Chapter 5

'Having to try' and 'having to choose': how IVF 'makes sense'

INTRODUCTION

In the previous chapter, two 'trajectories' were described in order to illustrate how the choice to opt for IVF is framed in relation to the disruptions posed by infertility, and subsequently how an IVF cycle poses its own disruptions. It was argued that descriptions of IVF itself as an 'obstacle course', a set of 'hurdles' to be negotiated, a 'way of life' and an experience that 'takes over' and that 'makes something of you' all are indications of the way IVF functions as a rite of passage. IVF is described as an experience structured by a model of achieved conception, in which determination to succeed, and faith in the enabling potential of technological assistance are definitive features of the trajectory established by the procedure. It has been argued that the importance of recognising these features of the experience of IVF must be contextualised within an under-standing of IVF as a process: a process which is entered into with expectations that change as the procedure 'takes over' and becomes a 'way of life'. Definitions of success and failure, for example, are changed in the process of undergoing IVF.

In this chapter, these features are explored in more depth, particul-arly in terms of their consequences for women's attempts to find a resolution to their infertility through IVF. Having established the ways in which the intensity of the technique imposes its own particular demands, and elicits particular strategies of coping and 'making sense', this chapter attempts to examine in greater depth the way the technique changes women's expectations and their long-term consequences. The chapter concludes with an evaluation of the technique seen in this light: in terms of the way IVF can be understood not only as a process, but as a rite of passage.

It is argued in the introduction that IVF is exemplary of the kind of emergent reproductive choice which has a very double-edged character. It typifies the kind of choice which is entered into with an expectation of enablement, and hope for an improved reproductive future through technological assistance, but which may well acquire a very different character once the process has begun. Presented as a simple technique, IVF turns out to be 'an obstacle course'. Chosen as a means of resolution, either by succeeding or being able to feel every effort was made, IVF generates its own momentum as a 'way of life', replete with new dilemmas and disappointments. Once IVF is chosen, new kinds of choices have to be negotiated, such as those presented by an ambivalent diagnosis or a 'partial success'.

That women can feel a sense of accomplishment and an empowering degree of determination in the face of the demands posed by an IVF programme is one side of the story. The other side is the cost that IVF imposes physically and psychologically. The pursuit of a 'miracle baby' may bring women closer to their partners, but it can also dominate their relationship and test their marriages to the point of near dissolution. Women may feel IVF 'made something of them' in a positive sense, but they may also feel disembodied, objectified, endlessly poked and proded or, as Meg Flowers put it, 'like a specimen on a table'. Coping with the failure of serial IVF attempts not only imposes severe emotional demands, but may ultimately lead to a profound experience of hopelessness. The hopelessness of never having children, the 'condition' IVF 'responds to', may be compounded by a hopelessness about ever coming to terms with this condition. If IVF offers resolutions to some women, it can also take away any hope of resolution for others. What IVF is seen to offer, in other words, *may be precisely what it takes away*. Nearly succeeding can be even worse than never coming close to success, as the hope has come even closer to becoming a reality, and the resulting loss is that much more devastating. Lost is not only all the effort of treatment, but everything about a woman's future a hoped-for success had promised, which can be a great deal indeed. In Frances Keating's words, 'It's your whole life you're talking about'.

Understanding the reasons why women choose IVF is thus essential to understanding their experience of the procedure. The reasons informing this choice, and the emotions which give rise to it, are the 'bottom line' informing the experience of undergoing IVF. It is all about hope: hope for success at each stage, hope for a resolution, hope for the future, and mostly hope for a child. Yet it is also all about failure. Even women who succeed have done so under the constant threat, if not several direct experiences, of failure. Even if they are 'successful', their IVF pregnancies literally embody this constant risk of failure, as they await each test with the same 'balance' of hope and preparedness for failure that shaped their experience of assisted pregnancy. Hence the language of miracles – miracle makers and miracle babies. After the experience of IVF, in which conception and pregnancy seem like an obstacle course, it is hardly suprising some women end up considering it a miracle that anyone ever gets pregnant at all.

'HAVING TO TRY'

One of the most striking features of the interview set is that in every instance women said they felt they *had* to try the procedure. Often this was stated in the same breath as the acknowledgement that they knew they would most likely be unsuccessful. In stark contrast with what women are left with in the majority of cases where they are unsuccessful, the ways that women enter into IVF were uniformly described in terms of 'having to try':

> I think when you have been trying for so long and you really want it you are going to try everything you can think of, that you've heard of that will do it, you know. . . . So we think it's only fair if you've tried everything and I've tried everything. . . . [We] both think that we should both do all we can, to see if it works . . . and I think well if I don't try am I forever going to be thinking if I had done? So I'll just keep trying. I mean at least I'll know in myself that we have tried everything and if it doesn't work then eventually we might accept it, but I feel I've got to try every possibility. As I say, if you really want it, you've got to try everything you can. You daren't give up on the first attempt. If you really want something, you have to go for it. I think you are willing to spend as much time as there is if you really want a baby. . . . I suppose there will still be loads of people that have had [IVF] suggested but who have said no, can't be bothered with that. But I'm not like that. You either go out and get it or you sit on your backside and leave it.
>
> (Jeanette Ives)

In this statement, the feeling of 'having to try' is repeatedly stated. It is composed of several elements. At one level, it expresses sheer determination: if you really want something, you will do whatever you can to get it. In addition, there is the feeling that you might look back at a future date and feel regret for not having tried everything. Noticeably in this extract, a clear distinction is made between people who do not opt for IVF and people who do. Jeanette Ives strongly categorises herself as a doer, a seeker – as opposed to someone who 'can't be bothered' or who sits on their backside.[1] She sees herself temperamentally as someone who does not give up easily, although she agrees that even she might give up eventually. Such a statement shows a clear awareness of the difficulty of IVF, the fact that not all women would chose it, and the determination to succeed that so thoroughly characterises the experience of IVF. The feeling of 'having to try' is both powerful and unhesitating. It is the feeling of 'having to try' which creates the feeling of 'having to choose' IVF.

The essence of this statement is articulated by Pauline Harding, who already had one child, and wanted another child both for herself and her partner, and for her son to have a sibling. When asked about her first response to IVF, she answered: 'It was just another way to have a child, so I said yes', adding 'At least I've tried, that's how I feel, at least I've done my best'. In a sense, the 'decision' to opt for IVF is precluded by the pre-existing desire to have a child. If the procedure is seen as the only way to realise this desire, then there is no decision, no 'choice'; the answer is a foregone conclusion.

For many of the women interviewed, the 'choice' of IVF presented itself in the form of the clinic's opening in October, 1988. As many of them lived nearby, and the local papers ran announcements about the clinic, a 'choice' which may have been lurking in the backs of their minds, or 'on hold' for whatever reason, suddenly surfaced and became immediate. Frances Keating describes her 'decision':

> When the clinic opened in October, there was a big splash in our local paper, [and I thought] haah, let's have a go! As soon as [my husband] came home I showed him that and we made our decision, well it's either your decorating or it's – because we'd just moved in, you see. I mean [my husband] says, well the choice is yours, *well there wasn't a choice*, I mean I just had, I had to have a go, for my own peace of mind, because you never, if you don't you're always saying well if only I'd had a go perhaps it would have worked?

Frances Keating's statement that 'there wasn't a choice' indicates well the paradoxical nature of 'choice' in the context of IVF. On the one hand, a choice was made. On the other hand, it is described as an inevitability: a foregone choice, as it were.

Frances Keating was one of six of the women interviewed who already had children (30 per cent), and among the three of those (15 per cent) whose children were adopted. Having adopted two children had partially enabled her to come to terms with her infertility, but this situation changed with the opening of the clinic. She continues:

> Mind you, we'd forgotten, we'd said alright, once we'd got the girls, let's just get on with it, accept that we're not going to have any and we can't get IVF on the NHS, let's just be done with it, and we'd accepted it pretty well until the clinic opened and then you go, ah! I've got another chance. I mean you've got to take it really, you've got to have a go, which is what we decided.

As this statement makes clear, she had more or less come to terms with her inability to give birth to children, had adopted children and had decided to 'get on with it', until the clinic opened nearby and thereby presented a new option for treatment. Yet, after two un-successful cycles, in which 'everything was fine', but a pregnancy did not result, coming to terms with the situation and attempting to just 'get on with it' became much more difficult. In the following account, extreme measures are considered as a way out of this dilemma:

> If it's not working for you you've got to come to a stop, you can't keep doing it, you can't drain yourself to rock bottom physically and emotionally as well as financially. There's got to be a time when you think, right, let's do something for us now, we've tried it. That's what I'm going through at the moment, I'm saying to myself, alright, we've tried it, I've done this, the dream that I'd always wanted to do is try. Alright, it hasn't worked, I've got to get on with my life now. . . . But it's ever so hard . . . you still never give up the wanting to have a baby . . . I don't know if I'll ever give that up . . . the actual wanting, the need, the desire to have a baby. . . . I mean we've resigned ourselves to the fact that we were always, we were never going to have children, never be able to have a natural born child. . . . But I don't think, even now I always think to myself, if I've come a day late kind of, wonder if I've done it? So you never forget it, I mean you have your monthly periods so you cannot forget it, I don't think you can ever give up while you're still having your periods

properly and everything, you never give up. 'Cause I even thought up to a month ago, why don't I have an operation and get rid of the lot, be sterilised, and that'll *stop* the wanting. . . . I thought if it's *gone*, it's *finished* that's the answer to *stop* it. But then I think to meself, well if I do that I know what's going to happen. Next week somebody's gonna bring something out and I could have done it! Can you understand that? You're pulled by your emotions both ways. . . . How do you find a happy medium to cope with it all? You never win. You can never have peace of mind. I mean that's just the way I feel about it, I know I will never settle.

As this description demonstrates, and as was noted above, what women look to IVF to provide *may be exactly what it takes away from them*. In other words, attempting IVF may be seen to be essential in order to feel that 'everything possible was done', all routes were tried, and no options were neglected. Even when they know they are likely to fail, many women who choose IVF do so in the hope that at least they will not look back later in life and wonder what would have happened if they had tried it. If they cannot be certain of the outcome of IVF, in terms of whether they are successful in giving birth to a child, at least they can hope for the certainty of knowing they did everything possible to succeed.

Yet, as Frances Keating's dilemma demonstrates, this is precisely the certainty that IVF takes away. From an uneasy but functional ability to 'get on with life' pre-IVF, she describes a shift into a 'no-win' position of indefinite irresolution: 'I know I will never settle'. She is without even hope of a resolution, feeling caught in a kind of Catch-22. Like the field of achieved conception itself, her future has become technologically dependent. She has considered extreme measures, a hysterectomy, to put an end to her distress. But even this will not provide a sense of 'resolution', because she fears the kind of newspaper headline that brought her into contact with IVF to begin with: a description of a technique she would 'have to try'. What if she comes home and finds the local paper running a feature article on a brand new technique which could enable someone like her to have children? Which would be the worse regret, to regret having a hysterectomy or to regret spending years of her life torn in two? She is faced with imponderables. Her 'choices', as she sees them, are both unsatisfactory, and she feels she 'can never have peace of mind' and that she knows she 'will never settle'.[2]

Frances Keating describes an attempt at IVF as a kind of dream come true: 'the dream that I'd always wanted to do is try'. By trying she could have her 'chance', her bid for 'a natural born child' of her own. In addition, even if she failed, she would at least know she tried everything, and would be relieved of the fear of looking back and wondering what might have happened if she had tried IVF. But this longed-for peace of mind eludes her, in the aftermath of IVF, which has left her bereft of consolation.

This theme of having to try IVF in order to feel they had at least reached 'the end of the road' was repeated again and again in the interviews:

> Well I think you feel you've got to try it. It may not work, but if that's the only thing that's left for you, you've got to try it. . . . I didn't want to feel in a few year's time, oh I wish I had tried that, you know, I had the opportunity and I didn't take it, I wish I had. I felt as if I might regret it, later on.
>
> (Mavis Norton)

> I don't want to get to menopause and feel I haven't tried everything.
>
> (Beth Carter)

> Yes [it is definitely worth trying IVF] because then you can live with yourself knowing that you did everything you possibly could, there was no other option open to you. . . . I think to know we've done everything in the end would have helped, would have helped to come to terms with it, because otherwise you would always have wondered had you gone through with it would it have worked.
>
> (Susan Doyle)

> I think that the decision that I felt was that if IVF was the only possible means then that was the avenue I wanted to go through to have our own child.
>
> (Meg Flowers)

> It's nice that there is somewhere you can go . . . that you could go down and have a couple of tries so you know like later on in your life you could think, you know, yourself, well, I've tried, I have really tried, I wanted a baby, I wanted a family, we have tried, we've given it all we can and they at the hospital, they've done all they can for us, like it's better than thinking well we might have been able to have a family if we had went and had treatment, if we had went such and such, do you know what I mean? You don't want to have that doubt there, at least you give a shot, you know.
>
> (Sara Yates)

As these speakers explain, IVF is sought not only to provide a child, but to provide a resolution to the uncertainty created by infertility. To 'know we've done everything' is sought as a means to 'come to terms with it'. The knowledge that 'you've got to try it', even though it 'may not work' is seen as a protective measure against 'doubt' or 'regret' in the future. Such fears are often correlated to the onset of the menopause, at which point a woman's fertility is seen to have ended.[3] The feeling that 'you don't want to have that doubt there' is thus an important motivating factor in the choice to undergo IVF, because then *even if it fails*, at least the knowledge that 'everything' has been tried will be some comfort.

Even women who expected the technique to fail often felt that at least trying would give them peace of mind, as Jennifer Young explains:

> I don't think I expected it to work, actually, I went in with a very negative attitude . . . but I felt we owed it to ourselves to give it a try.

These and the many other similar statements throughout all of the interviews emphasise the necessity of attempting IVF in order to come to 'the end of the road', and to ensure no avenues of possibility are foreclosed. The forcefulness of this logic is clearly apparent in the imperative to choose IVF expressed by many speakers in response to questions about their decision to undergo treatment. Invariably, this was not a complex decision; it was simple and obvious, so much so as to not even be a 'decision' or a 'choice' at all, but more of an inevitability. If there was a chance, it had to be taken. If there was hope, it had to be pursued:

> I think it sort of keeps you going to know that there is a chance. And if there is a chance you take it. The options are there, if you don't take them it is your own fault really, you can't look back and say if this had happened, we have tried, we have done everything possible to make it work.
>
> (Stephanie Quinn)

> It's not all a bed of roses, but if it works it's a bonus and it's better than nothing. It's better than no choice, it's better than being told last January that that's it and that would have been it totally, at least I have got a chance, albeit slim. There's a chance, and I think of it that way.
>
> (Catharine Lewis)

IVF 'keeps you going' because it offers a chance, the only chance of success. Likewise, as Susan Doyle put it, 'it is worth every minute because of the hope that it gives you'. In stating that IVF is 'your only chance' or 'your only hope', however, is a suggestion that keeping this hope 'alive' by opting for the only chance available is an important end in itself.[4] Again, the importance of 'making progress forward' in life is emphasised, as in the case of the descriptions presented earlier of how infertility renders women's futures tentative. Knowing that everything possible has been done, knowing that there is still hope, there is still a chance is initially seen as far preferable to the finality of being told there is nothing to be done. Later, some finality, or boundary is desired as a means to reach 'an endpoint' to the cycles of disappointment and failure. Again, it is the contradictoriness of the emotions and desires involved in IVF which are apparent here.

HOPE AND DETERMINATION

That keeping hope alive is important in itself again must be seen as a cornerstone of the entire IVF experience. It is what keeps women going through the arduous treatment cycles and is the source of their determination to continue. For this alone, for the hope that it gives, and the feeling that there is still something that can be done, which is being done, which they have chosen to do, rather than doing nothing, women unanimously recommended IVF when asked what they would recommend to other women in their position. As Mary Chadwick states:

> I would never ever put somebody off IVF. I would never say – oh, don't bother, it's pointless, it's useless, it doesn't work, because you see the results – it does work, and you've just got to be one of the real lucky ones for it to work . . . literally it's the luck of the draw when it comes to IVF. . . . As I say, I would never put anybody off going for IVF, because you've just got to use every option that's open to you.

Here, a belief in the technique in general, 'it does work', overrides the fact that the technique fails for the majority. This is explained as 'the luck of the draw'. In such a perspective is evident the forfeiture of a certain kind of control of ones future; as Mary Chadwick states 'you have to try' IVF, but 'you've just got to be one of the real lucky ones for it to work'. No amount of trying harder will ensure success, however important trying as hard as you can may be. It is like a kind of gamble or roulette. Hence, on the one hand, IVF is sought out as an enabling technology, yet on the other hand it is perceived as subject to a kind of random element no amount of assistance can mitigate. This is very similar to the situation of the ambiguous diagnosis, where the ability to produce quantities of sophisticated medical information does not add up to meaningful knowledge. The promise of technological enablement is not always realised. It is the *hope* it promises, as much as what it can actually provide in the way of a child, which is the reason it is chosen. In fact, dependence upon technological solutions is often *dis*abling, rather than the reverse. As Mary Chadwick continues, in a statement which runs directly counter to that offered earlier:

> Years and years ago, if couples couldn't have children, they just couldn't have children, because there is so much known about it now that I often wonder, if we hadn't started going to fertility clinics right from the beginning, would we have not been so uptight, pressurised, um, be more relaxed in trying to have a baby, whereas you're looking at temperature charts, the time of the month . . . and that's a pressure in itself. I mean we made light of it, but there's still that pressure . . . you're thinking in two week spans.

On the one hand, the 'hope it gives you' makes IVF a desirable opportunity. Yet this hope is also acknowledged to be disabling in its substitution of one 'tentative future' (infertility) for another (IVF).

It is this feature of the IVF experience which leads some women who fully endorse the technique also to state that it 'only makes life more difficult'. Given the disruptions produced by IVF, it is not surprising many women end up wondering whether they might not have been better off never having attempted it to begin with. In a set of statements which ran counter to their endorsements of the technique, many women were outspoken about its drawbacks. Having felt they 'had to try', many women none the less wondered whether having done so only left them worse off.[5] As Ellen Brown observed, 'it is a lot down the drain'. Other women expressed similar misgivings:

> IVF only makes life more difficult. . . . I would have had to accept it a long time ago if it weren't for IVF. At twenty-eight I could have either gone for adoption or accepted my situation so

I'd be five years down the line towards that and getting on with my life. Now you're in a better position to do that when you're twenty-eight than when you're thirty-eight. If you've missed all your career boats and burned all your career bridges because you've spent the last ten years chasing fruitless treatment you've actually missed out a lot on life.

(Beth Carter)

Going forward, determination is the most important component in the experience of IVF. Maintaining determination can be an end in itself, an accomplishment, an achievement against the odds in its own right. Struggling to maintain hope for success, faith in the technique and belief in the purpose of continuing on creates its own momentum. This goal-orientated mentality can be extreme. Kate Quigley stops just short of saying there is 'nothing she wouldn't do physically' to have a child:

If, I mean they've got a lady at the clinic and it's her twelfth attempt, and she's become pregnant on her twelfth attempt. If I were younger and if I had lots of money I would leave work and I think I would just have attempt after attempt . . . and if I had the time I think I would have the treatment sort of every three months until it worked. . . . I mean, you've got to put it in perspective, I mean up to a point you're prepared to go through anything to achieve a pregnancy, you are prepared to put up with the lot. . . . I think there's noth-, *I would go through more or less anything that they suggested physically*, you know, if they well if you had surgery or anything like that.

Emphasising she would 'go through more or less anything' to have a child, Kate Quigley expresses an intense determination to succeed. But looking backward, this determination may not seem to be such an accomplishment in itself. Often, it is a woman's age which ultimately prevents her from continuing IVF treatment. In other cases, lack of sufficient funds brought an end to treatment. The important point is that the determination to persevere along the 'road forward', the 'only avenue of possibility', can become such a 'way of life' that the likelihood of its being a dead end disappears from view. Indeed the possibility of this road leading to a dead end is precisely the possible eventuality which has to be so carefully managed, by balancing hope for success against the likelihood of failure, that *creates* the determination to continue.

Given that the women interviewed for this study were in the midst of treatment, it is not possible to provide data on their retrospective assessments of IVF. A follow-up study would be required to establish the nature of these assesments and the extent to which women's evaluations of their investment in IVF changed over time. Such a study, though beyond the resources of this project, would provide a valuable set of data regarding the 'other side' of the rite of passage involved in IVF. For example, one woman from the study who was interviewed on national radio approximately a year after the interview for this study, stated:

Interviewee: The first thing that any woman and her partner should think about when they feel that [IVF] is what they need is that *there are a lot of us who come away with nothing*. And although we may have our hopes fulfilled we may also have our hopes left unfulfilled and they should consider that one of their options is not to pursue treatment and there are many brave women who say I'm not going to take this any further, I'm going to stop now.

Interviewer: You say that but you yourself have been through several courses of IVF treatment.

Interviewee: Yes, I've started ten [IVF cycles] and I had my first one six years ago. I'm very grateful that I had the opportunity to do it and maybe, you know, the doctors will be able to improve the success rate of IVF because they were able to use women like me to learn, fine, but I'm not going to invest any more of my life in IVF because it hurts too much, it's too much of a payment to make and I'm not just talking about money. I'm talking about expectations, not pursuing your career, not having a holiday, all of those things that if you come to the end of the time and you haven't had your baby, you have to balance up what you've paid with what you've ended up with and I feel that I've paid my debt and I've ended up with nothing but I have accepted my infertility now.

(File on Four, BBC Radio Four transmission 05.12.89, transcript p. 14)

Explicitly framed in the language of investment, payments, and balances, IVF is seen to impose a high price. Although it is not claimed that the procedure is worthless, the speaker feels she has 'ended up with nothing' and her advice to other women is to take greater cognizance of this possible outcome. Likewise, although she does not say she felt exploited, she does refer to having been 'used' by doctors to improve their success rates, a comment which echoes many feminist criticisms of IVF as more important as a research technique than a form of therapy.[6]

The paradox of IVF is summed up in the statement that 'although we may have our hopes fulfilled we may also have our hopes left unfulfilled'. Similarly, although she states she is 'grateful' for having had the opportunity to try IVF, and has come to accept her infertility, the overall feeling conveyed is one of ambivalence mingled with regret. On the one hand she is glad she tried IVF, but on the other hand it was a costly investment which left her with 'nothing'. There is the sense of a double loss. Although she states she has come to terms with her infertility, the impression is not given that IVF made this any easier, which is what many women hope it will do, even if it fails. Instead, there is the sense that in addition to accepting her infertility, she has had to accept the losses she incurred through IVF, and that in this sense her losses were compounded, rather than eased, by pursuit of treatment. In addition to having lost 'the kind of life she would have led' as a mother, she has also lost the kind of life she would have led if she had accepted her childlessness earlier, and in this sense her losses have been doubled.

TENTATIVE RESOLUTIONS

The reasons for the apparent contradiction between her advice to other women and her own decision to undergo ten cycles of IVF can be seen to derive from many of the features of the experience of IVF presented in these chapters. Infertility is a condition which will lead some women to pursue every possible avenue of potential assistance, no matter how remote the chances of success may be. Once in the field of achieved conception, the procedure creates its own demands and thus a considerable amount of work, determination and endurance is required to continue treatment.[7] These strategies can involve complex mental 'self-management': an important component of 'living IVF' or of inhabiting the world of achieved conception.

It has been argued that this determination can become an end unto itself, as can any quest for an elusive goal. Moreover, it has been suggested that many of the features of the experience of IVF are only visible in retrospect. Going forward, women such as those interviewed are motivated by a strong desire either to succeed with IVF or to feel they have tried everything. IVF is seen as a road with two possible endings: success or failure. But neither is the 'end of the road' it is anticipated to be. Coming close to pregnancy, or achieving a 'chemical pregnancy', or even simply viewing her own 'fertility' through scans, can make it harder for a woman to accept her infertility than it might have been beforehand. Opting for technological assistance, seen to be enabling, can be disabling when technological assistance becomes technological dependency, and technological potential threatens a woman's own sense of agency.

One of the major ways in which this feature of the experience of IVF becomes apparent is in the way it brings a woman much closer to pregnancy, to her goal, and thus increases both the determination to continue and the desire for a child. Mary Chadwick describes the loss of a 'chemical pregnancy':

> One of the reasons I was talking to [a friend also undergoing IVF] on the Monday is . . . because I had gotten myself upset. . . . I looked through a photograph album and the last photograph . . . [was one that my husband] took of me in bed the day after [ET], and when I asked him why he'd taken that photograph he said it was because the grin on my face was so large, you know, it went from here to here, because the day before I'd gotten a positive result. Nobody can explain what a person feels when they say it's a positive result, and I just didn't stop grinning, but unfortunately I lost it. Getting over that was something else. . . . And when I saw that photograph, it brought it all back to me, that, you know, I *was* pregnant, even it being just a chemical pregnancy and that, you were told it was positive.

Even before a positive result two weeks after embryo transfer (a so-called 'chemical pregnancy'), many women 'felt pregnant' immediately after the fertilised embryo was 'transferred' into their bodies. I asked Frances Keating what it was like to see the embryos, which are projected onto a large screen before being implanted, adding yet another important visual dimension to the quest for achieved conception:

> Yes, oh, that was so emotional, that was, I didn't believe it would, but when I went in there for the embryo transfer, you're lying there on the bed, and they've got this screen, you know, this big television, and then quickly under the microscope and she says 'right, I'm going to bring them out now, now look quickly' because she wants to put them back because obviously she doesn't want to leave them there too long . . . and then all of a sudden

there they are and you *see* these little eggs that are dividing and well they are my babies 'cos they are my embryos, they're divided, they've just got to grow. And they are the actual start, it's the closest you've got to actually being pregnant, and oh I just burst out crying. Oh I just couldn't believe it. And when [the doctor] said there were three put back, you know, to me then I was pregnant, you know, I was actually pregnant, albeit it only lasted a week but I was actually pregnant, and you know that was just marvellous.

Actually feeling pregnant under these circumstances is hardly suprising given that the technique would appear to be one of literal impregnation. The tentativeness of this 'pregnancy', the fact that it is 'only' a chemical pregnancy – at once 'close' to pregnancy and pregnancy itself, again underscores the technologically-dependent nature of events in the context of IVF generally.[8] Neither is it suprising that such an experience would have the effect of increasing a woman's determination to succeed:

When I first attempted to get pregnant ... I think I was more philosophical about it, just, well, if I do get pregnant I do and if I don't I don't, and then sort of the longer it went on the more I realised that you know I really did want a family, and now I don't know what I'm going to do if I can't become pregnant. If I can't have a family, I really don't know how I'm going to cope with it. I decided that I'm not at all interested in my career anymore, in fact while I've been off this time, we've discussed it and I'm actually going to give up.

(Jennifer Young)

Yes, I mean I'd always, that's what I wanted, I always wanted children. I didn't want them desperately at the beginning, you know, like some people are absolutely, that's what they see as their role in life, and I mean I didn't feel that strongly about it, until we started going through all this, and I think when you are, when suddenly something is taken away from you, obviously you get very strong feelings about it.

(Christine Ingham)

In both these descriptions, a process of transition is noted, from a feeling of having to try IVF in order to feel that every option had been pursued, but not a feeling of 'desperateness',[9] to a feeling that the longer treatment continues unsuccessfully, the more focused the desire for a child becomes, to the point that, as Kate Quigley was previously quoted as saying, she 'would do more or less anything'. Notably, these women describe themselves as *not* 'desperate' initially, and as *becoming* 'desperate' *as a result of treatment*. This is the exact opposite of representation of 'desperate' infertile couples in the media accounts discussed earlier, in which the woman's 'desperateness' is what *drives her to seek IVF to begin with*. Likewise, whereas the media accounts describe IVF as *responding to* and *alleviating* 'desperateness', these statements suggest the reverse: that IVF is *the cause of* many women's increasing 'desperation'. Although IVF is ubiquitously celebrated as offering 'hope', it is this very hope which can *cause* the desperation it is said to alleviate. The search for a resolution through IVF, then, can be seen to create precisely the irresolution it was meant to eliminate.

It is this transition, from one side of IVF to the other, which is part of the 'passage' women may encounter undergoing IVF. It is a passage from one set of expectations, desires and experiences to another. But there is also an important difference. Classically, in ritual terms, a rite of passage involves the transition from one recognised social status to another (see Van Gennep 1906). This passage has been seen to involve a 'liminal' period of undefined ritual space between the one status and the other, which is seen as necessary for the shedding of one identity to make way for the acquisition of another in the ritually constructed space of ambiguity or social void of liminality (see Turner 1969).

In IVF, the transition is analogous, but different. The transition is internal, rather than public or collectively affirmed. It does not enter, but *begins* in a 'liminal space' of infertility, which is seen to *block* the transition from one social status to another. IVF is undertaken as a means to exit from this liminal condition (the 'limbo' created by infertility). Yet, IVF creates yet another liminality – a different kind of 'limbo'. The transition *out* of liminality is, thus, not provided by the 'rite' of IVF (unless, in the exceptional case, it succeeds). In other words, the 'rite' does not provide the 'passage'. Rather, the woman herself has to extricate herself from this rite of passage stuck in its liminal phase by an inward transition of some kind, such as coming to terms with her infertility and ending treatment. On the other side of such a decision, she indeed inhabits a different 'status', in the sense of having accepted an identity as either childless or with fewer children than she would like to have. A passage has thus been effected. If IVF has helped her to make this transition, however, it is not because of the technique itself, but because the procedure is something she felt she 'had to try' in order to reach a resolution. The point, of course, is that the IVF procedure has not necessarily made this resolution any easier.

DOUBLE-EDGED DETERMINATION

IVF is paradoxical in many respects. A sum of £2,000 is not a lot to pay for a child, if you have one. Even £20,000 may not be too high a price when it is something as intensely desired as a child of one's own. But either £2,000 or £20,000 is a great deal to pay for nothing. They are even more to pay for nothing minus the remainder of the investment, which includes not only the work, stress, disruption, physical pain and emotional heartache but everything a hoped for child had come to represent. In addition to 'nothing' there is the aftermath of failure, a 'debt' composed of a part of ones life that will never be 'repaid'. Like the wave of negative equity which succeeded the Thatcherite housing boom, IVF left many couples struggling to compensate for their overinvestments.

The cyclical nature of women's fertility, their menstrual cycles, that is, which is paralleled in the IVF cycle, also shapes the experience of treatment. Women describe the 'cycle' of hopes building up, the 'cycles' of coping with failure and the generally cyclical nature of their relationship to their infertility as well as the technology. Indeed, these are entirely conflated. This is emphasised by the measurement of time in terms of 'day one of the cycle' through to the last day, 'day X of the cycle', when a woman begins to menstruate. The descriptions of life's progression in terms of 'living in two week spans' or 'living month to month' constitute another way in which the 'way of life' of assisted reproduction becomes internalised, part of an identity, part of a world view. As time went on, over serial failed attempts, many women described their experience of IVF in terms of trying harder and harder while believing in it less and less. Mavis Norton uses the analogy of a 'wounded animal' to describe her hope:

> Because I think so much of it, it's a bit like a wounded animal. I mean if it's got somebody that loves it and is coaxing it and is saying get better and we love you and all of this and giving it a will, it will live. If it's deprived of that it will die. And I think the further you go on, the more resigned you are to the fact that it

probably isn't going to work. Because I was a lot more enthusiastic about it the first time than I am now.

Here, the reference to 'dying' not only indicates the extremity of the emotional experience of IVF, it also describes the central importance of hope remaining 'alive' in order for the will to continue to be sustained. The analogy to a 'wounded animal' describes the hope for success which initially spurred her own. After failing, the hope had to be nurtured back to strength in order for the 'will' to continue to survive. Yet, it has survived only to be tested again. As time goes on it is getting weaker: the desire to continue survives, but the will to do so fades. Resignation to the likelihood of failure replaces the initial enthusiasm about success. Yet, even this resignation does not protect against the continuing distress of failure. Ellen Brown describes losing heart:

I mean I have gotten past the stage of thinking it will work, and you know I am pretty sure it won't, but I mean you still get the disappointment, but I don't feel optimistic about it at all anymore.

When the hope, optimism and enthusiasm which carried women forward is lost, the will to continue diminishes too, creating doubts about the decision to pursue further treatment, and a greater readiness to accept that there is nothing to be done but accept their infertility, and get on with other things. Yet, even women whom the technique has failed and who feel they personally cannot continue, may express a continued faith in the technique itself. The belief in the enabling potential of technological assistance, often framed in terms of a more general belief in scientific progress, may well survive despite a woman's decision to terminate treatment. Frances Keating expresses this hope in relation to her daughter's reproductive future, in a telling intergenerational anecdote:

I mean when I listen to [my daughter] talk, she's on about, because of our going through the IVF, it would, I mean she was so upset when we failed with it, really was, and um, we've spoken, and she's said if I ever can't have children will I have to do this Mum? And I think to myself, well, maybe it'll be better for you, we're only in the first stages of it, I tell her, it's something new that's been brought in now, I said, but perhaps by the time you're old enough to have your own children, I says, and if you're unfortunate enough that you can't have your own children, perhaps there will be something for you. . . . I said there might be more perfection then, but I mean she's only nine, I says it might be better than it is now, because it's only just something that's been tried as a new thing. I said they're really, you know, they're not, it's not an everyday thing at the moment, is it? I mean it's better than it was ten years ago, I mean there were hints of it then, wasn't there, the first things that were being done, but now it's even better, and by the time she's older, it will probably be better still. There might be something else.

Annexing a belief in scientific progress ('there might be more perfection then') to hope for her child's future, this exchange precisely recapitulates the belief in natural science in the service of the natural family which is so definitive of public attitudes towards IVF. A similar view is expressed by Bob Newton:

I mean research is a funny thing, researchers can plod along for five years, ten years making only minute gains and then somebody has a flash of inspiration or something goes right and they take a great leap forward. It could be that in ten years' time we are not much further down the road of knowing about infertility, on the other hand in three weeks' time someone might discover a real breakthrough.

Many women expressed a similar faith in scientific progress:

I [have] a feeling of being really fortunate in being able to try this treatment, you know, to be able to have the treatment, you know, because it is very recent. I mean ten years ago, and really even five years ago, you couldn't, it just wasn't available. And in a lot of ways I feel really fortunate that I'm here at the right time in a way and that you know things have progressed amazingly.

(Christine Ingham)

They're learning all the time, and they're getting more and more successful.

(Ruth Levy)

Although occasional suspicion was expressed concerning the manipulation of embryos, IVF was uniformly endorsed as a worthwhile technique, despite having failed in the majority of instances, in which case the technique itself was praised, and seen to be improving, despite its unsuccessfulness for particular individuals. That IVF was 'recent' was even seen to enhance its desirability, adding a novelty value that created a 'feeling of being really fortunate'. This endorsement of IVF is thus part of an endorsement of science more generally, and is an affirmation of a belief in scientific progress as enabling, and in enabling technology as an outcome. Assistance in the realm of reproduction was endorsed in both these statements and in the frequently expressed praise for the clinic and its staff.

Such endorsements comprise an important component of the hope and determination which figure so largely in the experience of IVF. To attempt IVF, which is arguably a 'failed' technology as a result of its very low success rate, a certain degree of 'faith' is indeed required. This 'leap of faith' may be facilitated by a strong belief in scientific progress. This is evident in many of the extracts presented above, in which faith in scientific progress is shown not only to have influenced the choice of IVF, but to help in the acceptance of its failure, by creating a sense of having contributed to something larger than themselves.

MIRACLES OF NATURE

Somewhat more suprisingly, the naturalness of IVF was explicitly affirmed by several of the women interviewed:

> You hear all these things about test-tube babies and I think a lot of people think that it's quite an abnormal process, and I don't think we really appreciated what's involved. And I think we thought it was all a bit, um, clinical and – I mean I don't think we realised what a natural process it was, I mean it's only sort of emulating a natural process, it's just that it's sort of got outside interference and sort of done outside your body rather than inside it. . . . [W]e didn't realise it's as natural as it is.
>
> (Kate Quigley)

> I mean the end result will be the same as if it was all happening inside the body, it just happens outside the body, there's nothing peculiar about that. I mean it's like saying people shouldn't have kidney transplants and things like that, you know, because that's not natural . . . I mean I don't see it as any different from any sort of medical intervention at all for anything. I mean obviously if you get into the realms of trying to create a superbaby by two parents that are geniuses or something, then obviously that's an entirely different thing, but I don't consider them in the same

breath anyway, I don't see it, I mean I think it's going to become much more common anyway.[10]

(Christine Ingham)

This affirmation of the 'naturalness' of IVF is consistent with the infamous plasticity of ideas about 'the natural', and their ability to be readjusted even to circumstances which patently contradict this claim. On the other hand, if these ideas are considered to be symbolic, rather than literal, then the message is coherent. This message, after all, is that IVF is only 'giving Nature a helping hand'.[11]

At the same time, IVF is still considered a 'special' way to conceive. Although not seen as 'unnatural' in the sense of being immoral or abnormal, IVF is seen as 'miraculous' by many. Indeed conception itself comes to be seen as 'miraculous' under any circumstances, given how many obstacles there are 'naturally' to its occurring. In this way, the model of achieved conception produced in the context of assisted reproduction, such as IVF, comes to define conception more generally. The 'miracle' of assisted conception is conflated with the 'miracle' of natural conception in a manner which suggests the ways in which modes of 'making sense' particular to the field of assisted reproduction have the potential to become definitive of reproduction more generally. That 'nature' ever succeeds *without* a helping hand is as miraculous as when it succeeds in the context of assisted conception. According to this definition, every baby is a 'miracle baby':

I mean that's how I see it, it's a total miracle anyone ever has children once they're pregnant. You read the books, so much can go wrong, pages of all the different things that can go wrong at different stages.

(Christine Ingham)

I mean it's a miracle anyway when anybody has a child, but it just seems to be an even bigger miracle I'm trying to achieve, and as the old saying goes, impossible things take time and miracles take even longer.

(Meg Flowers)

Do you remember that programme on TV[12] where they showed you right from the beginning what was involved in conception? Fantastic it was, they actually showed you everything, it was as though they'd just dropped a camera inside a woman's body to see what caused them to conceive. And at the end of the programme they said it's a wonder anybody does get pregnant, so many obstacles to it.

(Peter Levy)

When you sit down after five years of effort and the specialist says to you well you fall into the unexplained category, that's I think the key to it. We do not know. It's like saying every generation thinks it knows everything and that there's not much more to find out, but we really don't know what happens when a sperm meets an egg, or why sometimes it fertilises and sometimes it doesn't.

(Bob Newton)

In these extracts, the way in which the experience of IVF changes understandings of conception are apparent. From a normal, natural sequence which is clearly understood and scientifically legitimated, conception becomes a 'fuzzy area'. From a simple causal chain of events, conception becomes a badly designed process that hardly ever works. This is the point of view of reproduction which is defined within the field of assisted conception: nature needs a helping hand. According to this view, it is a miracle indeed that nature even gets off the starting blocks without technological assistance.[14] If natural conception and pregnancy are 'miraculous' considering the apparent odds against their occurring unaided, then IVF is an even bigger miracle in its confirmation of the potential for technology to subsume this function successfully. 'Miracle babies' are the result of IVF, not of 'nature'. They are the definitive offspring of assisted conception, their very existence making manifest the enabling potency of technology.

The contradiction between IVF being seen as 'natural', in the sense of 'just doing what nature would do anyway', and IVF being seen as a 'miracle' is functional. It allows IVF to be perceived at once as 'miraculous' and as 'normal'. It allows for 'nature' and the artifice of technological assistance to reproduction to be reconciled. Indeed, they become one, analogous to one another. Nature is like a badly designed machine, and technology is just doing what nature does anyway. Natural processes, technological intervention and the 'invisible hand' of human scientific agency are thus unified.[15]

This view of assisted reproduction also enables women and couples who participate in IVF programmes to feel part of a much bigger process, that of scientific progress. As noted earlier, opting for the enabling potential of IVF is also an endorsement of the enabling potential of scientific progress more generally. Hence, individual failure can be understood as a 'success' in so far as it makes a contribution to 'greater understanding' or improving the technique. There is the possibility of a vicarious participation in something greater than the individual, the couple, the IVF team or the clinic.[16] Failed IVF can potentially be viewed in almost sacrificial terms, whereby, for example, a mother expresses a hope that her own failure will at least lead to a potentially improved situation, should her daughter need reproductive assistance.

CONCLUSION

So far in this part of the book, various features of IVF as a 'way of life' have been explored with a view to emphasising how the experience of IVF is 'made sense of' and inhabited. This experience is discursively constructed at the level of popular culture within media representations such as those discussed in Chapter 2. It is also structured internally by the parameters of the clinical discourse of assisted reproduction. Finally, it is defined by the individuals who participate in IVF programmes and formulate their own 'lived understandings' of what is occurring, and their own ways of making sense of the procedure.

Within this constellation, there are both overlaps and disjunctures. As the clinical construction of reproduction is one in which it appears as an obstacle course, beset by potential sources of failure, and in need of assistance, so too do women describe the technique of IVF as an obstacle course, and conception as so beset by risk of failure it is a 'miracle' anyone ever conceives at all. Similarly, as the media construction of IVF emphasises the disappointment suffered by couples whose lives have not progressed along conventionally established routes, so too do women and their partners describe this as a major source of distress. As the clinical discourse constructs reproduction mechanistically, so too is this how many women come to think of it themselves, becoming experts in the 'nuts and bolts' of conception. As the media portray IVF as scientific progress in the service of happy families, so too do women describe their perceptions of the technique.

Yet, to note these concordances between the discursive construction of IVF, its popular portrayal in media accounts and women's own descriptions of the experience of IVF is not to assume there is a seamless continuity between them. Most important among the disjunctures between popular representations of IVF and the experience of it is the overemphasis upon the reasons women choose it, and their expectations going into it, to the exclusion of the ways in which these can change and come to look very different further on. As has been noted, IVF can take away precisely what it is anticipated to provide: a means of resolution, a feeling that everything has been tried, and hope for a means of completion. The willingness to undergo IVF is structured by expectations which are themselves transformed by the intensity of the procedure, leaving women with only their own ingenuity and determination to make sense of the altered situation in which they find themselves. Though this can be satisfactorily accomplished, the costs may well be unexpectedly high and the options are limited as to how one comes to terms with being on 'the other side' of IVF. Looking forward, and going forward, can be motivated by a very different picture from that encountered with hindsight, when making the best of failure may prove far more difficult than initially envisaged.

It is for this reason that the experience of IVF has been examined here in terms of both the particular mentality it requires, and the way in which it can be seen as a rite of passage. Both these terms refer to the unexpected way in which IVF 'takes over' and becomes 'a way of life'. The mentality of IVF is comprised of a number of factors. It involves a careful balancing of hope for success against preparedness for failure. It involves tremendous determination to succeed. It requires a particular attitude, as well as particular kinds of labour. This in turn sheds light on how the difficulties presented by IVF are negotiated, how and why the technique is described as 'taking over', and, especially, how this mental adaptation comprises part of 'living IVF'.

The idea of a mentality or mindset to IVF is also useful to emphasise the very paradoxical components of what is required by it, and the habituation to these conditions the procedure often entails. IVF presents contradictory demands: to hope enough but not too much; to try your best but realise it is a gamble; to make sense of the unexplained; to believe in miracles. It is a technique that is both simple and complex, 'natural' and 'achieved'. Through IVF a woman can come closer to preganacy, 'see' her 'fertility', be 'impregnated' and become a 'mother' or 'pregnant', by which means she can both feel 'more fertile' and more acutely the pain of infertility. IVF can 'reassure' that 'there is nothing wrong' despite there clearly being 'something not quite right'. Failure and success in IVF terms are both relative and absolute, dependent on the outcome 'in the end'. But one of the most difficult questions involved in IVF is when the 'end' will be. IVF is a choice, but not a choice. It is a resolution but not a resolution. It 'makes something of you' but 'leaves you with nothing'. It is something women recommend but wish they had not done. IVF is described as a wonderful opportunity, and as only making life 'more difficult'.

That IVF 'takes over' is thus not merely logistical. To negotiate a successful passage through IVF requires physical, emotional and psychological 'self-management'. This in turn explains how IVF functions as a rite of passage, involving the search for a resolution as well as the attempt to achieve reproduction with the aid of technological assistance. The important feature of a rite of passage is that it involves transition. One possible transition is from the inability to reproduce successfully to the production of a 'miracle baby'. But this is the exception.

The other desired transition going into IVF is a reproductive resolution: an end to reproductive 'limbo'. It is an important argument of the analysis of IVF presented here that the technique itself can make the attainment of a resolution more difficult. Although this is not necessarily the case, the interviews suggest the ways in which women's needs and expectations of the technique *change over the course of treatment*. Going into IVF, either a resolution or a baby is described as the expected outcome, leading to a security of mind that one or the other will result. On 'the other side' of IVF, it is evidently possible that neither outcome will have manifested itself, thus leaving a woman without an apparent means of satisfactory conclusion.

It is also argued that this feature of IVF is, like the world of achieved conception more generally, a product of technological dependency. IVF is described as a 'hope technology' because it is the hope it promises, as much if not even more than a 'successful' outcome, which leads it to be seen as a desireable option, even when it is expected to fail. The problem is that although 'the hope it gives you' makes IVF seem 'worth it' at the outset, the hope is not enough indefinitely. This hope, like so many aspects of the IVF experience, is double-edged, both enabling women to continue and dis-abling them from reaching an endpoint of treatment.

Ultimately, women are left with what they invested in the technique to begin with. They are left with the courage to put themselves to the test, the determination to carry on against the odds and the resourcefulness to find resolutions and make meaningful sense out of whatever situation they eventually find themselves in. Women who successfully give birth to IVF babies will feel in their relationship to those children the sense of achievement that child literally embodies. Women who are unsuccessful can feel a different sense of achievement, of having tried everything possible and having determinedly persevered to the extent of their endurance or their emotional, physical or financial limits.

Justifying IVF as a procedure in terms of women's 'desperate' desires to have it, or representing IVF as technology's answer to the plight of the 'desperate infertile woman', must be seen as inadequate legitimations. Women who choose IVF because they needed to try everything, as the women interviewed unanimously claimed, are not only expressing a desire for children, but a desire for a resolution. In so far as IVF rarely provides a child, and not only fails in the majority of cases to provide a resolution, but can take away the means of doing so in the process, it can only be seen, at best, as a partial response to women's needs. That *it is not possible* 'try everything' is the realisation with which many women terminate their relationship to IVF.

It is important to repeat that the interviews were exclusively conducted with women who had a very high estimation of the technique. The evidence for this was substantial. The amount of praise for the technique and for the clinicians was striking. Women frequently expressed their gratitude, good fortune and 'luck' in being able to undergo IVF, *even when they failed*. Even after devastating experiences of failure and loss, none were critical of the technique. All gave it a ringing endorsement and stated they would recommend it to other women. Not all women would respond in this way, nor would all groups be so homogeneous in their collective endorsement of the technique, however ambivalently this was at times expressed.

Both the uniformity of this response, and its generally affirmative tone may be due in part to the fact that the women interviewed were either in the midst of IVF treatment or had been until very recently. In this context, such endorsements can be appreciated as instrumental, enabling and functional. To think otherwise under these circumstances would indeed be almost perverse. Moreover, even among this group of women, who on the whole expressed an extremely positive assessment of the technique, a noticeable degree of equivocality and doubt is apparent.

Despite giving the technique an endorsement, some women also stated it would have been easier for them if it did not exist, or if they had never tried it. Despite coming to terms with their situation ably and determinedly, many women were also frankly outspoken about its costs. Although able to feel a sense of accomplishment and achievement, many women also felt enormously drained both physically and emotionally. Although highly appreciative of the support they received from others, they also expressed concern about the ways in which the technique created tension and stress in their relationships, including those with family, friends and colleagues as well as their husbands and children, if they had them. Although none of the women interviewed articulated statements of regret on the whole, many expressed reservations, even in the midst of treatment, and all were candid in their admission of how much more the procedure affected them than had been anticipated at the outset.

The argument here is not that 'the real truth' of IVF lies beneath a superficial veneer of naive or self-affirming endorsements of the procedure. It is rather an argument that the 'truth' of IVF, like the conception models discussed in Chapter 1, is multiple and contradictory. The argument is that women's experiences of IVF, in their own terms, are far from simple. They are composed of feelings and perceptions that are equivocal and ambivalent, positive and negative, empowering and disempowering. These paradoxical dimensions of the experience of the IVF procedure are fundamental to many of the ways of making sense of it described in these chapters. Balancing hope for success against awareness of the likelihood of failure, believing in the technique against the odds, creating a sense of achievement out of serial losses, and the many similar challenges posed by the demands of the procedure are all characterised by at least dual, and often conflicting, impulses and desires.

Such a claim is, none the less, sufficient to argue that media representations of IVF are incomplete, and that medical justifications of the technique as responding to women's needs are, at best, partial. However, such an argument is limited for several reasons. To begin with, it assumes that preferable representations or justifications would be 'more accurate'. Since representations are not neutral or objective to begin with, this is an argument with a limited purchase, though not one that is without its importance. Moreover, the argument here is precisely that there are substantial obstacles to providing an 'accurate' representation of IVF, given that women are likely to change as a result of going through it, and that what may seem 'worth it' at the beginning may not appear so at the 'end'. In addition, experience is not the only measure of a technique such as IVF. Though a crucial component in any assessment, it is not sufficient in itself. 'Experience' as such is not accessible, rather a set of representations of it are. These are mediated by several factors, and constitute here a set of transcribed statements collected from interviews conducted with a particular group of women in the midst of treatment. At the very least, experiences are continually re-evaluated, and a follow-up study to this one, with the same group of women, concerning the same set of experiences, would undoubtedly contain different versions from those recorded here. Since experience is inevitably contradictory, it is never 'complete', and it is always subject to multiple readings both by those to whom it is communicated and those to whom it belongs.

These chapters too are representations of the experience of IVF. Like other representations, they are purposeful, selective and constructed in accordance with particular aims. The findings presented here confirm those of other researchers who have investigated women's experience of IVF. Like Crowe's (1985) study, the material presented here confirms the socially constructed nature of the choice to opt for IVF. This is not only indicated by the very noticeable importance of normative social conventions in the articulation of the choice to opt for IVF, but also by the largely uncritical 'investment' in dominant cultural belief systems such as scientific progress. Like Williams's (1988a and b) Canadian studies, the attitude of determination, 'It's Gonna Work For Me', has been found to be a major factor accounting for why women continue treatment in the wake of serial failure. In addition, the interview material for this study indicates the importance of a search for resolutions, accounting for why the technique is pursued *even when it is expected to fail.*

This finding is also relevant to Koch's (1990) Danish study in which the information about failure rates 'did not matter' (1990: 225, emphasis removed). Indicated by the present study would be that a successful outcome, in terms of a 'take-home baby', is not the only goal motivating the choice of IVF to begin with. This, then, extends Koch's argument as to why IVF does not constitute an 'irrational choice', given its high failure rate, but instead must be understood as part of a specific 'rationality'. Koch argues this rationality is based on the desire for a child, and the fact that IVF may be the only potential means of achieving this, *regardless* of the likelihood of failure. A desire for a reproductive resolution, *regardless of the outcome of IVF*, could be seen as complementing this argument.

In all of these studies, an attempt has been made to reconcile women's experience of IVF with what would appear to be the inexplicability of women's desires to undergo a largely unsuccessful, costly and demanding form of reproductive assistance. To those features of the experience of IVF described by other researchers could be added here the difference between what IVF looks like going into it and the meaning it takes on later during treatment. In this sense, it might be suggested that a focus on the 'choice' alone is too static an account, to which a more processual or diachronic perspective is usefully added.

It is not a finding of the present study that one reason women opt for IVF is out of ignorance or misinformation, as is suggested by Klein's (1989) study. However, several features of Klein's study are confirmed. To the claim that 'IVF fails women', for example, can be added its failure to provide a reproductive resolution as expected. It would also be accurate to conclude, as does Klein concerning women who opt for IVF, that the women interviewed for this study do not see themselves as 'colluding' in the medicalisation of reproductive control. To the contrary, as has been indicated, the women interviewed for this study were, on the whole, full of praise for the clinic staff and the 'opportunities' afforded them by IVF.[17]

An important point here is that it should not be assumed, as critics such as Klein appear to do, that if IVF is understood as violent, painful and dangerous that women will decide to reject it. In descriptions of aspiration, women were explicit about acute levels of pain for which they often felt unprepared. In describing IVF as 'like running the Grand National with your legs tied together and wearing a blindfold' it is apparent women perceive it as physically dangerous and unlikely to succeed. In the description of aspiration as 'being stabbed in the belly' is evident an explicit image of violence. Such descriptions are not incompatible with continued treatment. They may even be evaluated positively, in the sense of 'having tried everything', perhaps even to the point of heroism. Similarly, an awareness by women that they are being 'used' by doctors to 'increase their success rates', or to learn how to 'improve their technique' is not necessarily considered a disincentive.

The evidence presented in these chapters suggests that women's experiences of IVF do not conform to any simple conclusions in terms of critically assessing IVF. Like the way the experience of IVF itself is described by women who have undergone it, so too must the assessment of women's experiences acknowledge the often paradoxical and contradictory dimensions of what is occurring in that encounter.

However, it was not an aim of this study to take a position 'for' or 'against' IVF, as has been the case in much of the feminist discussion of this technique. By situating the conception narratives derivative of the world of achieved conception in relation to the broader cultural values which define it, my aim instead has been to draw similarities with other models of conception from other cultures, and to note the usefulness of this perspective in relation to the ongoing development of anthropological models of kinship, parenting and procreation. In this respect, it is clear that one of the most important features of the accounts presented here is their complex negotiation of the values of progress, choice and technological enablement. As such, these conception narratives index wider features of the cultural context of which they are a part. The dilemmas expressed in the context of IVF, in particular the desire to 'embody progress' and thus become a conduit of both 'natural' and scientific continuity bespeaks a particular kinship universe. It is to this universe and its distinctive constellations that the final chapter is addressed.

Chapter 6

The embodiment of progress

INTRODUCTION

As noted in the introduction, this book is organised around a contrast between the historic importance of certainty about the 'facts of life' within anthropological accounts of conception models cross-culturally, and the uncertainty now characterising the 'biological facts' of human reproduction in the context of achieved conception. This contrast is provided as a means of establishing a refractory perspective on the givenness of these 'natural facts' in relation to both kinship and gender theory. In this final chapter, I begin by locating this refraction in the context of parliamentary debate of the Human Fertilisation and Embryology Bill, which reached its culmination during the period of fieldwork for this study, and which comprises an elaborate debate about 'the facts of life' not entirely dissimilar to those pursued within the 'virgin birth' debates in anthropology.[1] By so doing, I propose to explore the workings of 'the biological facts of human reproduction' in terms of their cultural importance to contemporary British culture. In turn, this perspective 'refracts' on the importance of a specific model of 'the facts of life' in the history of British and Euro-American anthropology.

As noted in Chapter 1, Schneider critiqued the anthropological study of kinship for having been based on a presumed genealogical model of relatedness, which itself reflected the 'folk models' of European culture (1984). Similarly, in her account of the 'virgin birth' debates, Delaney argues that a Judaeo-Christian model of monotheistic creation informs the monogenetic concept of paternity assumed by anthropologists over much of the past century (1986). Mary Bouquet adds specificity to the claim that genealogy is a 'folk European' artefact by arguing that it is in some respects particularly

British, or even English (1993). Uniting these perspectives is the view of Yanagisako that it is the givenness of the 'biological facts of human reproduction' which has structured anthropological models of both kinship and gender (Yanagisako 1985, see also Yanagisako and Collier 1987). Finally, the givenness of these 'natural facts' has been linked to hegemonic operations of 'the natural' within Euro-American society by a range of commentators, developing what has become a key strand in feminist anthropology and feminist cultural theory (Franklin 1991b; Haraway 1989, 1991; Strathern 1992a and b; Yanagisako and Delaney 1995).

By invoking the contrasting conception models that structure *Embodied Progress* as a whole, my aim is to contribute to this debate about the 'biological facts' which have structured so much British and Euro-American social theory by exploring one specific context of their elaboration. In a suggestive, rather than conclusive, manner I offer here an account of how these 'facts' can be read as broadly symbolic not only of the generative power of a sequence of bio-logical events (egg meets sperm makes baby), but of the generative power and authority of scientific knowledge. I am suggesting that 'genealogy', in the form of life's continuity, or life's progression, not only does service for models of kinship, but for models of knowledge. I closely follow Strathern, whose arguments have focused on the role of ideas of the natural in the constitution of culturally specific ways of knowing, in this interpretation (1992a and b). Historically, my reference is the importance of 'conceiving' as both an epistemological and a procreative act.[2] Here, I offer an additional exemplification of these conceptual processes, though approaching them from a different angle.

As the last three chapters have illustrated, the world of achieved conception produces an unfamiliar perspective on 'the facts of life'. Whereas these 'facts' are deemed so obvious that no one could possibly be ignorant of them in the context of the 'virgin birth' debates (Leach 1967, Spiro 1968), they are far less 'obvious' in the context of IVF. Rather than being 'clear', in vitro fertilisation renders conception opaque. For every instance in which a sperm and egg unite to produce a pregnancy, there are many times more cases in which pregnancy does not result, and for these 'missed con-ceptions' there is no explanation. Much as it comprises a domain of elaborate expertise about 'the facts of life', in their strictest bio-logical sense, the experience of both couples and professionals in the context of achieved conception is inevitably one that foregrounds 'ignorance' of the 'facts of life'. At their most explicit, biological explanations of 'the facts of life' are revealed as *most* effective for explaining successful pregnancy: when a pregnancy is established, biology provides a causal explanation. These same explanations are *least* effective in the context of reproductive failure, in which all of the known causal determinants are present but a pregnancy does not occur. For such an eventuality, the technical term is 'unexplained infertility'.

Into the breach of explanation is inserted technological enablement. Sometimes, for reasons that are not clear, IVF can bridge the gap in the biological sequence leading to the production of pregnancy. Most of the time it cannot. Importantly, this failure does not destabilise the biological model: IVF is still considered to be 'giving nature a helping hand'. The result of failure is instead the renewal of hope. As the previous chapters illustrated in some detail, hope comprises a major component of the IVF experience. In the face of assistance to conception failing to produce the desired outcome, couples either give up hope for success and abandon IVF treatment, or they renew their hope and 'have another go'.

The inadequacy of the biological model of 'the facts of life' is directly reflected in the language of hope and miracles defining the world of achieved conception. It is a measure of how incomplete biological models are that when they are coupled with technological assistance and succeed, the result is a 'miracle baby'. Much as the comments of would-be parents and the professionals that assist them in the context of IVF emphasise the normalness and naturalness of assisted conception, they also affirm that there is 'something special' about the children born from this technique. These children are seen to embody the special efforts invested in their creation, both by their parents and by clinicians.

In turning to the parliamentary debates concerning human fertilisation and embryology, this language of hope and miracles takes on a further specificity. In this context, the hope expressed by women seeking IVF for a technological miracle to relieve the anguish of their infertility took on a prominent importance. Reference was repeatedly made to this hope, so much so that parliamentarians opposed to IVF explicitly commented upon its overvaluation. In the next section I offer a brief account of the role of 'hope for a miracle' in debates about the 'facts of life' with a view to examining in more detail the consequences of Euro-American 'ignorance' about 'the facts of life'.

HOPING FOR A MIRACLE

The use of 'hope for a miracle' to legitimate the procedure of IVF is not restricted to media portrayals of 'desperate infertile couples', and stories of happiness and hopelessness. Reproductive desire, annexed to faith in scientific progress, was also a key feature in much public debate concerning the new reproductive technologies in Britain in the 1980s. It served not only as an important, but in a certain sense as a uniquely privileged, form of evidence. In parliamentary debate of the Human Fertilisation and Embryology Bill, and accompanying media coverage, for example, accounts of the 'desperate' desire of infertile women and couples were frequently used as a form of witnessing, or testimony, in support of assisted conception.

The following, for example, is a typical extract from the parliamentary debates of 1989–1990 as a result of which IVF gained official state approval as a form of reproductive intervention, and became subject to governmental regulation via the Human Fertilisation and Embryology Authority. The extract is taken from the opening debate (the Second Reading) of the Human Fertilisation and Embryology Bill in the House of Lords, in December 1989, which occasion was of major importance in establishing the foundational arguments informing subsequent proceedings. The speaker is a parliamentarian who has been to visit an IVF clinic in Cambridge, where she met and spoke with a woman undergoing IVF. In the following passage, she describes this occasion in language that is immediately reminiscent of the generic conventions structuring the popular media accounts discussed in Chapter 2:

> IVF has seemed almost like a miracle for desperately unhappy couples who are able to undertake the new process. . . . I am speaking today because I have been able to visit the IVF clinic at Addenbrookes Hospital in Cambridge. . . . I saw one woman who is a senior midwife. She loves her work and is obviously dedicated to her patients, but until now she has had the experience of delivering babies day by day while unable to have one of her own. She has had two failed IVF pregnancies but is now in the 25th week of her third pregnancy and is expecting twins, if all goes well. She has to stay in bed in the clinic for a highly critical period of time just now, and probably for most of the rest of her pregnancy, but she said: 'It's all worth it – without IVF I would never have had the chance of having a child'.
>
> (Baroness Llewelyn-Davies, House of Lords,
> *Official Record*, 7 December 1989, cols 1023–4)

This passage is noticeably similar to the accounts of reproductive desire encountered in the media representations in several respects. The language of 'desperateness' and 'miracles' is used in the description of the relation between the individual woman and the promise of new reproductive technology. The extract typically describes the woman's needs and desires in the midst of treatment, indeed we encounter her at a 'highly critical period of time'. It thus describes the 'going forward' mentality described in the last three chapters. Despite two failures, IVF is still described as 'worth it' because it is the only 'chance of having a child'. The extract thus describes the *potential* of technology and the desire for a techno-logical miracle.

This description is also effective because it relies on eye-witness testimony. In this extract, Baroness Llewelyn-Davies describes how she has seen for herself the hope that IVF can provide. Her formal public testimony recounts the impact of having personally witnessed what IVF can offer. She has herself been convinced by what she has seen, and is seeking to convince others on the basis of her own experience. It is the experiential dimension to such images, in this case the experience of the woman described being amplified by the parliamentarian's experience of meeting her, which makes them so effective. The issues at stake are rendered more human, more meaningful and more poignant for their being depicted in this way, through the hopes and sufferings of another person rather than in the rarified and abstract language of ethical principles or moral duties.

Many parliamentarians, like Baroness Llewelyn-Davies, became similarly convinced of the value of IVF through visits to IVF clinics. These were arranged by Lord Jellicoe, a member of the House of Lords and the Medical Research Council, to enable parliamentarians to 'see for themselves' what new assisted reproduction techniques can offer. Similar eye-witness testimony was often referred to in debate, as in the extract above, as a conversion experience. Doubts were dispelled in the face of the immediate evidence of medical science in the service of would-be parents.

By definition, women who are attending the clinic are still 'living in hope' for a successful pregnancy. The clinic is the site of this technological promise and potential, *and it is this 'hope' which is the most important value signified by the image of the desperate infertile woman*. In this sense, the image is metaphoric: it stands for a belief in scientific progress and faith in technological enablement. It is a symbolic image of hope for an improved future, and of faith in the ability of medicine to alleviate human suffering. It is an image that powerfully unites traditional family values with faith in the power of science, technology and medicine to improve the human condition. In this sense, the image stands for much more than the woman herself. It is not only an image of individual needs, or even the collective needs of a group of similarly deprived individuals. Above all, it is hope that this description valorises.

It is very noticeable in the extract from Baroness Llewelyn-Davies that she has *not* seen the outcome of the scenario she describes. She has not witnessed a miracle, and her testimony is not based on having done so. What she has witnessed is *hope for a miracle* and *faith* in the capacity of medical technology to provide one. All she has witnessed is conviction, dedication and belief. That in her view this is sufficient grounds to be convinced of the value of a technology which she has not even seen be successful precisely demonstrates that success is not only, or even mainly, what it offers.[3] The most important feature of the image of 'desperate' infertile woman is the hope it signifies for the joy of a miracle birth. Here again, we encounter IVF as a 'hope technology', but this time in the context of the hope it *symbolises*. The hope of the individual woman described can function as a symbolic hope because it is so widely shared. It is not only *her* hope that is at issue, but the shared collective hope invested in the promise of science and technology. The effectiveness of such imagery is that it stands for instrumentality as an end in itself. *It is for this reason it does not even need to be stated whether or not this woman succeeds.* Her success is not what is at stake. It is her hope which is the important component.

Indeed, in the explicit way in which women's bodies became the hoped-for conduit for a technological miracle, it might even be suggested a religious comparison is not inappropriate. The kind of image invoked by Baroness Llewelyn-Davies is not only symbolic: it is *iconographic*. It is a *devotional* image. This woman (a dedicated nurse) has devoted herself to hope in a technological miracle. We bear witness to her devotion through her suffering, and also through her dedication. But importantly, we also bear witness to her *faith*. As she says herself, this faith alone makes her ordeal 'worth it'. It is this same faith with which scientists and clinicians 'devote' themselves to devising more effective means of repro-ductive management.[4]

The power of eye-witness testimony to the benefits of IVF played a crucial role in overcoming opposition to the technique, particularly from parliamentarians who opposed IVF on the grounds that it involved production of embryos that are not reimplanted. Especially for parliamentarians opposed to abortion, to which assisted conception technology was linked throughout the proceedings, the compelling nature of descriptions such as those provided by Baroness Llewelyn-Davies proved a constant source of annoyance. That such descriptions played a key role in parliamentary, as in wider public, debate was explicitly noted by more critical commentators. It was precisely the effectiveness of such imagery that was of concern to those who sought to challenge it. That such images, and their 'special place' in the argument was both noted and challenged in Parliament provides a measure of their disproportionate influence and persuasive capacity:

> The joy of those who achieve fertility or are able to achieve a baby through IVF has been described from all sides of the House. It is developing a special place in this argument.
>
> (Lord Kennet, House of Lords, *Official Record*,
> 7 December 1989, col, 1028)

This comment, also taken from the critical Second Reading in the House of Lords at the outset of parliamentary consideration of the Human Fertilisation and Embryology Bill, attests to both the 'special' character of the experience of 'those who achieve fertility or are able to achieve a baby through IVF' and the frequency with which such descriptions were employed in parliamentary debate. In the face of such evocative and emotive imagery, it is difficult to voice opposition: who would want to deny this hope or prevent this joy?

At one end of parliamentary debate, then, is the concrete image of the 'desperate' infertile woman who has invested her hopes in technology, and the couples who have experienced the joy of successful pregnancy. At the other end of the spectrum is what the technology itself represents. In the following triumphant plea for legalising embryo research, Sir Ian Lloyd makes explicit the basis for faith in scientific progress, and the wide scope of the hope it offers:

> The discovery of DNA, the very blueprint of life, is certainly awe-inspiring, and when the full map of the human genome is known, probably within a decade, we shall have passed through a phase of human civilisation as significant as, if not more significant than, that which distinguished the age of Galileo from that of

Copernicus, or that of Einstein from that of Newton. Its political significance is almost beyond our comprehension. We have crossed a boundary of unprecedented importance. . . . There is no going back. . . . We are walking hopefully into the scientific foothills of a gigantic mountain range. Hitherto, man has had no option but to come to terms with a serious burden of genetic impairment, but now he can look ahead, perhaps a long way, to its eventual elimination. . . . For us to forswear the assistance which science can provide in modifying that code to the advantage of the human race would be an indefensible abdication of responsibility. It would cross the portcullis of this place with a most sinister and destructive bar.

> (Sir Ian Lloyd, House of Commons, *Official Record*,
> 23 April 1990, cols 96–8)

Although this extract concerns the use of new genetic technologies, the reference is also to IVF, in so far as an important justification for the use of IVF was the proposed implementation of gene therapy via this technique.[5] Two primary groups of 'afflicted persons' were foregrounded in arguments based on experience. One was of the infertile, and the other was of carriers of genetic disease who could be helped to have healthy children via IVF, such as those referred to here.

However, the most important component of this extract is again the reference to hope: of 'walking hopefully into the scientific foothills of a gigantic mountain range'. The hopefulness expressed towards technology is given much fuller explication in Lloyd's description. It is, for example, given a moral imperative. Not to pursue scientific inquiry is described as 'indefensible', 'sinister' and 'destructive'. Scientific progress is described as inevitable: 'there is no going back'. There is no stopping this advance, we cannot 'close the doors' on the 'frontiers of human knowledge', to do so would not only be 'unenforceable', but would 'merely inflame curiosity', claims the speaker. The will to know is described as an intrinsic human need and an essential moral good.

The hope and faith invested in technological progress is here proclaimed in its most expansive and exalted form. The entire future of the human race is seen to be at stake. The imagery of scientific pioneers entering new terrain, the foothills of 'the gene age', whose significance is 'almost beyond our comprehension', is again almost mystical. The image is of scientific knowledge lying in wait to be discovered. There is no sense of choice or options within this depiction of scientific progress: it is as eventually inevitable as it is morally imperative to proceed forward.

Interestingly, this counter-image to that of the 'desperate' infertile woman-martyr also introduces her saviour in the form of the heroic scientific pioneer. On the one hand is the devotional woman figure (*mater dolorosa*) beckoning miraculous technological impregnation, whilst on the other is the forward-marching scientific pioneer devoted to the cause of fathering invention. Both images have powerful symbolic resonance within Judaeo-Christian doctrines of divine creation. It is man's fate to have eaten from the tree of knowledge and been burdened with mortality. It is woman's fate to suffer in childbirth and to be subservient to patriarchal authority. As the potency of the Father and the Holy Ghost were realised through the vessel of Mary's womb in the miraculous conception of Christ, so are women's bodies in the context of IVF the symbolic repositories of a profound faith in the moral and historical imperatives of scientific progress.[6]

Similar religious symbolism attends the use of foetal imagery which, it has been suggested, make of the fetus a Christ-like figure. As Faye Ginsburg has noted in her analysis of foetal symbolism in the context of the American abortion debate, 'the aborted fetus becomes a sacrifice offered for the redemption of America' (Ginsburg 1989: 107). Similarly, as Barbara Duden has argued in the context of the abortion debate in Germany, the fetus becomes a 'public sacrum', a sacrifical object of worship symbolising a wide array of social ills (1993b). A kind of religious mystery surrounds the tiny, perfectly-formed fetus in its private inner sanctum which has been converted into a powerful source of overdetermined symbolic rhetoric by right-to-life campaigners. As Rosalind Petchesky argues:

> 'The foetal form' itself has, within the larger [American] culture, acquired a symbolic import that condenses within it a series of losses – from sexual innocence to compliant women to American imperial might.
>
> (Petcheskey 1987: 268)

In Britain in the 1980s, the joy and hope of those who sought to achieve a miracle baby through the power of science and technology served as a similar condensed image, not of losses, but of potential gains. Through the mobilisation of a potent form of reproductive imagery, the promise of scientific progress was affirmed and celebrated.

That such religious parallels appear in the context of evocative imagery concerning reproduction is hardly surprising given the importance of beliefs about conception to cultural accounts of human origins or genesis.[7] As anthropologists have been quick to discover elsewhere, beliefs about conception are inseparable from questions about what it is to be human, how a human comes into being and the 'miracle' of this creation. In the long history of western scientific accounts of generation, from Aristotle's writings on the subject in the fourth century BC through the contributions of William Harvey in the seventeenth century and up until the present, conception has been inseparable from metaphysics and cosmology (Dunstan and Sellers 1988). There is no reason to assume that increasing knowledge about 'the facts of life' over the past two centuries has entirely dispelled this legacy. To the contrary, the celebration of the joy of miraculous births in the British House of Commons in the 1980s wholly corresponds to the 'awesome mystery' of life's creation and the transcendent cultural values with which this potency has long been symbolically associated.

In the iconographic image of the 'desperate' infertile woman, and the equally important symbolic figure of the 'miracle baby', are evident not only a devotion to the ideals of scientific and technological progress, *but their capacity to be embodied*. Through IVF, science and nature are unified in an act of pro-creation. This is a critical interface. Symbolically, this union and its 'fruit' not only signify, but actualise, the potency of natural science in the service of the natural family. Where there was no family, technology has enabled one, through an act of miraculous creation, at once the product of nature and of science. The 'miracle baby' is both the 'fruit' of knowledge, and of the germline: it embodies their unity, it confirms their potency, and ensures their continuity.[8]

It is in this way that the desire for assisted conception functions as a sign in public debate. Far from being a literal description of the experience of IVF, in which hope plays a far more complex and less enabling role, the truncated description of the hope and joy of infertile couples is the repository of condensed signification referencing collective cultural hopes and faith. The joy occasioning the birth of a miracle baby is a sign: a sign of embodied progress.

FAITH IN PROGRESS

Like the 'virgin birth' debates described in Chapter 1, the parliamentary debate about human fertilisation and embryology in Britain in the 1980s was defined by a structuring absence. In both the 'virgin birth' and in the parliamentary debates, this absence was of 'correct' knowledge of the 'facts of life'. For anthropologists debating 'virgin birth', the presence of an absence was seen to require explanation in terms of core features of social organisation and cultural belief. The same can be said of the parliamentary debates. Here too, an absence of complete knowledge reveals the presence of core principles of social and cultural life. Both the traditional family values invoked by the spectre of infertile couples' disenfranchisement from society, and the cultural value of belief in scientific progress and technological innovation, emerge as the direct referents of incomplete knowledge of 'the facts of life'. It is *because* these facts are incomplete that faith in scientific progress is a moral necessity, and once they are more complete ('once the complete map is known'), the value of hoped-for progress is confirmed.

An important implication of this similarity is that the meaning of 'the biological facts of reproduction' is not simply literal. Not only are the 'facts' of biology symbolic in the sense outlined by Schneider, as symbols of 'diffuse, enduring solidarity' or kinship ties. They are also symbolic of possession of a particular form of knowledge, which offers a particular access to truth. This explains why questions of knowledge and truth were so important to the 'virgin birth' debates. The 'biological facts of human reproduction' not only signify the 'truth' of reproduction, they signify *the power of science to determine this truth*. Moreover, this knowledge is attested to by its instrumental power, that is, its power to generate or to create. In this sense, an implicit analogy links 'biology' with *knowledge of* biology: they are both endowed with generative power. I suggest this has important implications for the metaphor of genealogy.

Put another way, the argument can be restated. In the event of reproductive failure, or infertility, no one argues that it doesn't really take an egg and a sperm to make a baby. The response is that a sperm and an egg *should* create a baby, and that technological assistance can *help* them produce a baby. In other words, the biological function of fertilisation is seen as capable of being assumed technologically. That is what the world of achieved conception is all about. Similarly, when IVF fails, which it does most of the time, the response is not to abandon the attempt to assist conception, but to improve the technology to achieve a better outcome. Technology can provide what nature fails to deliver: it can bridge the gaps, make the connections, and assist nature in doing what it should have done 'naturally'.

The point is that 'nature' and 'technology' in the context of IVF are not only commensurate, but substitutable. Just as IVF clinicians 'learn' from nature how to improve their techniques, so 'nature' can be improved by scientific and technological assistance. Much as the domains of science and nature have been positioned in historic opposition, it is equally true that the development of science depended upon the invocation of nature as a separate, lawlike, mechanical realm of phenomena *which was compatible with scientific representation and intervention*. In this sense, they became the same thing.

Schneider points to the specificity of the modern western model of 'nature' when he argues that the Yapese do not assume that people and pigs reproduce in the same manner. It is the assumption that people and pigs *do* reproduce in the same manner which enables Darwin to 'borrow' the analogy of kinship to describe nature as a system, thus instantiating the modern biological definition of nature, or life itself, as a single unity. Darwin defines nature as a system of consanguinity, just as Morgan does, in proposing a distinction between descriptive and classificatory kinship, as Strathern points out. IVF extends this 'loan' yet again: instrumental knowledge can be substituted for biological function in the context of reproduction, still one of the most 'naturalised' domains of human activity. Moreover, this instrumental capacity can be seen as 'just like' nature, as confirmed by the 'natural' and 'normal' birth of a child as a result of their coupling.

It is the creative potency of this substitution, the ability for science to assume and thus become part of the reproductive process, which is signified by the denomination of such a birth as miraculous. Possession of 'accurate' (modern biological) knowledge of the 'facts of life' is thus not simply about the 'literal' truth of physiological events leading to conception, for possession of this form of knowledge signifies something much more than the literal truth itself. It signifies a power of instrumentalism, and indeed faith in its enabling capacity. 'Nature' is not only knowable through techniques of observation, representation and intervention, but it is thus appropriated as an extension of these techniques, to become instrumentalised. This is what the absence of accurate or complete knowledge of 'the facts of life' in the context of assisted conception reveals by effecting an immediate shift into the language of hope, faith and miracles – all of which refer to the power of science and technology to transform 'natural facts' into culturally-desired outcomes, including progeny.

POSTMODERN GENEALOGY

The conflation of scientific knowledge with life itself, which is the conflation I argue IVF materialises, is evident in Sir Ian Lloyd's elaborate defence of scientific progress. Like DNA itself, scientific knowledge has been passed from generation to generation, from Copernicus, to Galileo, to Newton and to Einstein, he suggests. The discovery of DNA offers to extend this progress into 'the very blueprint of life'. This promises the 'eventual elimination' of 'genetic impairment' which he describes as a moral necessity: 'For us to forswear the assistance which science can provide in modifying that code to the advantage of the human race would be an idefensible abdication of responsibility.'

In the midst of a legislative effort to establish 'human fertilisation and embryology' as juridical territory, this statement expresses not only the capacity for science to 'assist' nature, but the imperative for it to do so. Any other option, in Lloyd's view, would be no less than 'sinister'. As in the context of IVF, the analogy used by Lloyd is of the 'assistance' science can offer, in this case to 'modify' human heredity. The suggestion is of 'assisting' genealogy.

Assisted conception already anticipates the direct modification of heredity, in so far as it comprises a form of assistance to intergenerational transmission. The 'eventual elimination' of genetic 'impairment' would require more elaborate 'modifications'. These are already becoming available in the form of genetic therapy for 'inborn errors of metabolism' such as cystic fibrosis. Often, gene therapy is proposed for severe childhood diseases, and the same admixture of hope for success and preparedness for failure characteristic of would-be parents in the context of IVF is likely to be the experience of families of children who are candidates for genetic assistance. Assisted genealogy will become an increasingly widespread kinship dilemma.

This study offers a perspective on this dilemma, both at the level of how it is experienced, and in terms of its implications for understanding 'what kinship is all about'. I have argued that the parliamentary debates concerning human fertilisation and embryology can be seen as a context in which the reproductive hopes, desires and joys of infertile couples functioned not only as evidence of the good that new reproductive technologies can achieve, but in addition that these hopes symbolised the broader cultural value of belief in scientific progress. I have suggested that the belief in scientific potency in the context of new reproductive and genetic technology is increasingly seen as commensurate with the generative power of life itself, so that they are substitutable for one another.[9]

Looking back at the 'virgin birth' debates, it is clear that the concern with 'the biological facts' of human reproduction was also a concern about a specific *form* of knowledge, not just its content. Implicit in this concern is the status of anthropological knowledge as itself scientific. The ability of anthropologists such as Malinowski, Leach or Spiro to interpret the conception models of the Trobrianders or the Australians in terms of deep structural, or hidden psychological, or structural-functional meanings accessible to the trained observer articulates a belief in science as a way of knowing. In the same way that the Judaeo-Christian model of paternity expresses a particular view of the power to create, the modern biological model of the 'facts of life' expresses a particular view of the power to know.

One of the meanings I propose here for postmodern kinship theory is the sense in which it is no longer possible to assume this particular view of the power to know unproblematically. This is a contested claim, and much of the resistance to postmodernism derives from the view that it is anti-scientific, relativist, or even nihilistic. There is a widespread sense of anxiety that 'abandoning' the claim to be scientific will be accompanied by a loss of evaluative standards. I suggest that these standards have already been lost: their bases in a particular worldview have already been made explicit, and this is itself an effect of increasing cultural diversity (See Marcus 1995). Anthropology is in a unique position to turn such insights to its advantage. It is not the case that evaluative standards will be lost. They will simply change, as they have already done.

Kinship theory has also to be 'after the biological facts' for the simple reason that biology itself continues to change, as it has always done. For Malinowski, the possibility remained open that certain cultures do not 'know' the causal relation between coitus and pregnancy. This was the verdict of Ashley Montagu, whose assessment Malinowski described as the most fully scientific ever achieved. By the time of Leach and Spiro's dispute, the possibility of 'ignorance' had been rejected, and the 'facts of life' were assumed too obvious for anyone not to know at some level. In a sense, for Leach and Spiro, this knowledge was itself naturalised as so self-evident as to preclude non-recognition by any human group. For Schneider, Weiner and Delaney, modern biological knowledge of the 'facts of life' was simply irrelevant to the kinds of questions about culture anthropologists needed to ask. For these same theorists, it was the importance of biology *within* western culture which required attention, as a means of challenging ethnocentric and gender bias – a task to which Strathern's work remains the most comprehensive response.

As anthropologists have turned to the question of the significance of biology *within* Euro-American society, however, the task of defamiliarisation has also been aided by biological science itself. It is a direct result of advances in reproductive biology that parliamentarians in Britain spent many hours debating the meaning of 'mother', 'father', 'conception', 'fertilisation' and the legal status of embryos stored in liquid nitrogen tanks across the country. This process itself denaturalised 'the facts of life' by specifying precisely how they could, or could not, be 'assisted'. Far from being *semper certa*, reproductive biology has increasingly become a site of contestation.

In terms of kinship theory, then, the 'genealogical grid' once assumed to be a fixed point of reference, authenticating both a set of 'biological facts' and the power of science to produce accurate knowledge of them, can no longer be assumed *even on its own terms*. Not only is it now visible as an historic artefact of 'folk European' models of relatedness, but it has been rendered artefactual *within biological science*. The advent of transgenic organisms, trans-species hybrids, patented immortal cell lines and genetically modified strains of plants, bacteria and livestock augers a major departure from the Darwinian genealogical grid.

As contemporary Euro-American, and increasingly global, kinship debates, the many redefinitions of genealogical connection at issue in debates about biodiversity, the human genome project, genetic screening or molecular evolutionary studies can usefully be approached as both post-natural and postmodern conception stories. It is not necessary to resituate the genealogical grid: it has already been relativised. We are already 'post' the modernist model of consanguinity: it has been geneticised, technologised, instrumentalised,

commodified and informationalised and reproduced as virtual sequence data alongside the genomes of mice, dogs, worms, yeast and
fruit-flies. Neither can 'science' be unproblematically assumed to be
extra-cultural any longer.[10] Likewise, 'kinship' can no longer be
defined as a question of 'natural', 'biological' or 'reproductive'
facts, as these criteria are no longer 'given' in the context, say, of
paternity disputes over artificial life forms. The anthropological task
lies in understanding what kinds of cultural phenomena such disputes
comprise, and what an anthropological perspective on such questions
looks like. Postmodern kinship theory is one way to describe such a
project.

CONCEIVING THE FUTURE

The population described in this study are also 'post' the modernist
model of the 'facts of life'. Although some, such as Rabinow (1992),
argue that assisted genealogy (or conception) represent the apo-
theosis of modernity – its intensification rather than transformation,
I suggest this would be a more accurate description of the route in
to IVF than the route out. The will to take action, to do something,
indeed to try everything is the classically modern mentality out of
which the choice to opt for IVF emerges. Belief in progress, and hope
for improvement are the defining features of the quest for conception
in the context of IVF. Coping with failure by renewing hope for
success might well be described as exemplifying a modernist attitude
towards the possibility of an enhanced future through ingenuity and
innovation.

  For most of the people who encounter the world of achieved
conception, however, it is eventually necessary to abandon this hope,
to abandon a belief in progress and to come to terms with having
failed to achieve their goals. Moreover, one of the features of this
experience I have tried to show in some ethnographic depth is the
flipside of the 'hope that keeps you going' in the way that this hope
can become disabling. It is none the less also a finding that many
people who fail at IVF continue to believe in the potential of the
technique to improve over time, as some of the comments recorded
in the previous three chapters attest. However, the postmodern turn
does not require abandoning belief in progress, nature or scientific
authority, it merely requires the acquisition of an additional layer of
doubt concerning their effectivity.[11] It is the specific admixture of
continuing belief in the tenets of modernity, and increasing un-

certainty about precisely these goals which is the sense of the postmodern condition I would claim describes most people's experience of IVF.

The dilemma of 'embodying progress' thus describes the kinship situation derivative of technological assistance to reproduction and heredity. This will continue to expand in social, cultural, political, economic and moral significance as consanguinity becomes increasingly geneticised, medicalised and instrumentalised.[12] Much as forms of human connection may continue to be naturalised, the simple determinism of 'natural facts' and traditional biological models of conception are already outdated in such a context. Helpfully, this anachronisation of the 'biological facts of reproduction' is complemented by the possibility of rediscovering their significance in the conceptual apparatus of anthropology itself, now newly available as a cultural field in its own right. This combination of circumstances offers a greatly expanded scope for kinship study, which might usefully be redefined as the study of vital signs and their connections, including those that connect bodies of knowledge with the peoples who are constituted in and through their many agencies and constraints.

Notes

INTRODUCTION

1 This study both contributes to and draws upon the recent anthropological work addressing kinship in the context of new reproductive technologies. In particular, it extends arguments developed out of collaborative research on this topic funded by the British Economic and Social Research Council, published as *Technologies of Procreation: Kinship in the age of assisted conception* (1993).

2 See Squier (1994), for an account of the specifically British fascination with 'babies in bottles' in the post-Darwinian era.

3 For a discussion of the 'enterprise culture', see Abercrombie and Keat (eds), (1991). See also Chapter 2.

4 For discussion of the importance of conception beliefs in anthropology, see Jorgensen (1983). See also Delaney (1986, 1991) and Inhorn (1993). For a discussion of contemporary conception narratives, see Franklin and McNeil (1993); McNeil (1993); Franklin (1990a, 1991b 1992, and 1993); Martin (1991).

5 I am indebted for clarification on this point to Corinne Hayden, whose interpretations of Strathern's arguments strongly influence my own. See especially Hayden (1997).

1 CONCEPTION AMONG THE ANTHROPOLOGISTS

1 A growing body of scholarship has addressed 'the making of the modern body' and the specificity of western scientific understandings of biology, including gender and reproduction. See Gallagher and Laqueur (1987); Laqueur (1990); Jordanova (1989); Schiebinger (1987, 1989); Strathern (1992a).

2 For a discussion of the return of genetic essentialism in late-twentieth century Euro-American culture, see Nelkin and Lindee (1994); Franklin (1991b); Hubbard and Wald (1993).

3 Yanagisako's paper was delivered at a panel devoted to Schneider's work at the 1985 annual meeting of the American Anthropological

Association. My thanks are due to the author for sending me a copy of her paper at the time.

4 Key sources on the 'virgin birth' debate include: Austen (1934); Barnes (1963, 1964, 1973); Delaney (1986); Leach (1967); Merlan (1986); Montagu (1937); Mountford (1981); Malinowski (1916, 1927a, 1927b, 1929, 1937); Powell (1956, 1969a, 1969b); Roheim (1933); Rentoul (1931); Sider (1967); Spencer and Gillen (1899) and Spiro (1968). For case studies of conception theory in New Guinea and Australia, see Battaglia (1990); Biersack (1983); Eyde (1983); Jorgensen (1983a, 1983b); Hiatt (1971, 1978); Kayberry (1939); Montague (1983); Mosko (1983); Poole (1983, 1984); Haüser-Schaublin (1989); Strathern (1988, 1995); Wagner (1967, 1983); Williamson (1983); and Weiner (1976, 1978, 1979, 1988). Correspondents to *Man* include: Derret (1971), Dixon (1968); Kayberry (1968); Leach (1967, 1968); Montague (1973); Powell (1968); Douglas (1969); Schneider (1968c); Wilson (1969); and Spiro (1968, 1972).

5 The relationship between anthropology and scientific method in Malinowski's work thus relies on an admixture of conjunction and separation. On the one hand, anthropology is seen to be in need of becoming more scientific. Yet, scientific facts 'pure and simple', such as those from the biological sciences (e.g. consanguinity) are argued to have no place in sociological sciences. At one level, then, science provides a common ground for sociological and biological *methods*; yet at another level, they should remain separate undertakings. See further in Nader, 1996: 259–261).

6 An important gender difference thus characterises Malinowski's approach to 'biological facts': while paternity is, in a sense, de-biologised, maternity remains a primarily biological relation. Indeed the nurturing component of the maternal–child bond is itself subsumed within a bio-functionalist model of inherent human needs that it is the purpose of society to meet. Hence, for Malinowski, maternity is to biology what paternity is to culture.

7 For additional comparitive accounts of conception in Melanesia, see Jorgensen (1983) Mosko (1983), Strathern (1988, 1995: 42–4). See in particular Haüsser-Schaublin (1989).

8 By mapping generative agency among the Trobrianders in this manner, Malinowski reproduces a familiar Judaeo-Christian model of genitorship as singular. That there is a 'genitor' at all among the Trobrianders, or whether it can be seen as singular, are questions raised by both Annette Weiner (1988) and Carol Delaney (1986) to which I will return below.

9 The importance of conception models to the entire matrix of social organisation is repeatedly underscored by Malinowski. As Weiner goes on to argue in her reworking of Malinowski's work on Trobriand society, such a view clearly positions reproduction at the heart of social organisation: conception beliefs form the basis for kinship and exchange, which in turn comprise the elementary social, political and economic relations.

10 While attentive to the racism and ethnocentrism of anthropological constructions of 'primitivism', Leach overlooked the cultural import-

ance of a closely related discourse of primitivism within European biological science, specifically embryology. A suggestive parallel to the discourse of primitivism structuring questions of ignorance or rescience of the 'facts of life' among the Trobrianders and the Aboriginal Australian peoples, is the importance of the notion of the primitive within embryology. As debates in the British Parliament at the time of this study made clear, the emergence of 'the primitive streak' (the early backbone) in the developing embryo proved an essential mark or line denoting early human origins. See Haraway (1976) for insightful discussion of early twentieth-century debates about embryology.

11 Hence, although Leach was very eager to compare western *religious* beliefs to those of the Trobrianders, he avoided any such comparisons to western *science*. The argument, for example, that western scientific beliefs are also cultural, and map, if not the metaphysical relation between gods and men, the relations between mankind and transcendence (in the form of scientific truth) was not of interest to Leach. It was of interest to his colleague at Cambridge, Joseph Needham, and later Robert Young – who argued that the debates surrounding Darwinism in the late nineteenth century precisely concerned the 'replacement' of 'god' by 'nature' (1985). In turn, students of Young's, such as Maureen McNeil, have provided detailed documentation of the importance of spirituality to natural scientists, such as Erasmus Darwin, Charles's grandfather (1987).

12 According to the OED, 'parthenogenesis' is originally a biological term, first appearing in the mid-nineteenth century, and later used by Darwin in *The Origin of Species* (1859). The use of the term 'parthenogenetic' to mean 'born of a virgin' is introduced by Tylor in his *Primitive Culture* (1871).

13 Interestingly, Spiro here implies that within the Trobriand spirit-child belief, there is no model of genitorship – a point which would seriously undermine his argument that the repression of knowledge of paternity represents the wish of the male child to be his own genitor. To sustain this conclusion, Spiro would have to argue that the Trobrianders repress not only knowledge of physical paternity, but of any notion of genitorship whatsoever.

14 Here again, Leach demonstrates his reluctance to consider modern biological science alongside the 'higher religions' as 'variations on a single cultural theme'. Again returning to his colleague Joseph Needham, it is no coincidence that Needham's interest in science as a cultural system in China led on to his compendious history of embryology, in which branch of European science the proximity of religious and scientific imagery is especially pronounced (Needham, 1975; see also Dunstan and Seller, 1988; Dunston 1990).

15 The 'magical' substitution proposed by Spiro is thus to replace actual, but repressed, knowledge of human (paternal) genitorship with 'another genitor', the spirit-child – which consciously held explanation masks a patricidal fantasy of auto-genitorship. However, as noted above, this assumes an isomorphism at the level of the notion of a 'genitor' in both cases. As Delaney (1986) notes in her critique of the 'virgin birth' debates, such an assumption leaves unexamined the cultural organisation

of generative agency, which may or may not allow for a notion of 'genitor' at all (as Strathern argues for the Hagen, 1988).

16 Returning to the theme of the links between science and religion foundational to modern biology, it should be noted that the cultural analogy of evolutionary theory – that life is like a tree – is taken from the Bible. As Mary Bouquet has argued (1994), the only illustration in Darwin's origin of Species (1859) is of an evolutionary tree, which he explicity compares to The Tree of Life in the Old Testament story of Genesis.

17 Schneider was profoundly influenced by the work of Talcott Parsons in his approach to culture, seeing it as a distinct domain of social life, somewhat in contrast to the models of culture deployed by many of the theorists influenced by his work.

18 Significantly, it was Thatcherism that brought Hall to this conclusion. No longer could politics be explained in terms of a model of ideological control that was either rational or class-based, he argued. The 'dominant cultural logic' didn't work that way: it was more diffuse, more unpredictable and more subterranean. In particular it was the popularity of Thatcherism among the working class which forced this turn-around within the British Left (or sections of it) to abandon the more economistic, class-based, and rationalistic models of ideology in favour of a more 'cultural' approach, within which politics, to use Hall's formulation, is more like a language (1988).

19 Two recent studies of conception models in contemporary American society offer suggestive parallels to Weiner's problematisation of generative agency. In her study of surrogacy, Helena Ragone provides a most intriguing account of 'Conception in the heart', relocating generative agency away from the biological events involved in fertilisation, and positing it instead in the parental desire to conceive. Strategically, this conception model repositions both parents as equal contributors in the generation of progeny, re-establishing an equality that is otherwise contravened by the unequal (biological) contribution of husband and wife in cases of commissioned surrogacy. In another example, drawn from an analysis of lesbian accounts of conception via self- insemination, generative agency is redefined as 'kinetic' rather than genetic – again providing a conception model inclusive of the bio- logically 'excluded' partner to procreative coupling (Hayden, 1995).

20 For excellent discussions of the origins and uses of paternity as a representation of genius, see Battersby (1989). For authorship, see Gilbert and Gubar (1979) and Rose (forthcoming). See also Franklin (1996) for a discussion of paternity and scientific knowledge.

2 CONTESTED CONCEPTIONS IN THE ENTERPRISE CULTURE

1 The 'British' government exercises power over the United Kingdom of Great Britain and Northern Ireland, which is commonly called Great Britain, or simply Britain. Technically, Great Britain refers to the unity

of England, Scotland and Wales. The United Kingdom properly describes the country as a whole, to which Northern Ireland (at that time all of Ireland) was added in 1800. I use 'British' to refer to the UK. I also move between 'British' and 'English', since this study was based in England and my main cultural concerns are with Englishness. It is, of course, important to note that 'English' and 'British' are not synonymous, and that this slippage is itself something of a contested practice, reproducing as it does the privileging of Englishness over the other national traditions out of which Britishness and the United Kingdom are constituted.

2 For accounts of 'Thatcherism,' see Hall (1988), Jessop *et al.* (1988), Cloke (ed.) (1992), Franklin *et al.* (1991), McNeil (1991). For the 'enterprise culture' see Keat and Abercrombie (1991).

3 The population of the UK is approximately 56 million inhabitants, of which 46 million live in England. By contrast, the US population is 226 million, according to 1992 figures.

4 Although assisted conception was expected to become highly profitable in England, as in other parts of the world, it has not, on the whole, proved so successful in business terms. It is instead the large pharmaceutical companies, such as Organon and Serono, who made the largest profits on IVF through their patent-protected monopolies on Clomid, Metrodin, Perganol and other drugs essential to the IVF technique. The far greater success of the pharmaceutical industry in making profits on IVF was epitomised by the purchase of Bourne Hall, Steptoe and Edwards' flagship enterprise near Cambridge, in the late 1980s by Serono, subsequent to the clinic's bankruptcy.

5 For an account of the development of infertility devices in Britain between the private and the public sectors, and for a critical account of their provision, see Pfeffer and Quick 1988.

6 Full details of the IVF procedure are provided in the following chapter. See also Fishel and Symonds 1986.

7 The *Warnock Report* stated that: 'It is better for children to be born into a two-parent family, with both father and mother, although we recognise it is impossible to predict with any certainty how lasting such a relationship might be' (1985: 11–12).

8 Although the clinic served a radically mixed clientele, only white couples agreed to be interviewed for this study.

9 This causes a certain amount of terminological confusion. In general, I refer to 'women', rather than 'women and couples' because this study documents women's experiences more than those of couples. However, where women considered 'the couple' as the patient, I have tried to make this clear.

10 For live birth rates resulting from IVF programmes in the UK, see the published *Reports* of the Voluntary, and later 'Interim', Licensing Authority (1986–91). This function was assumed by the Human Fertilisation and Embryology Authority in 1991.

11 See Klein (1989) and Klein and Rowland (1989) for an account of both the known and as-yet indeterminate hazards of the drugs and procedures used in IVF.

12   The advent of assisted conception in Britain, as in other countries, dramatically increased the incidence of multiple (more than two) births. The consequently elevated levels of perinatal complications, and their impact on already-stretched NHS resources, was one cause of concern. Equally draining was the impact of multiple births on would-be parents unprepared for the enormity of care required by three or more infants. For an account of the social impact of multiple births in Britain at the time of this study, see Botting *et al.* (1990). See also Price (1992).

13   Confidentiality was also discussed at the time of the interview, and pseudonyms for all of the interviewees are used in this book to protect the privacy of all those who participated in this study.

14   Studies by Crowe (1985); Koch (1990) and Sandelowski (1993) strongly support the findings of this study. For additional accounts of the experience of IVF, see Inhorn (1993); Lasker and Borg (1989); Lorber (1987, 1988, 1989); Modell (1986, 1989); Pfeffer and Woollett (1983); Williams (1988a, 1988b).

15   For accounts of the passage of the Human Fertilisation and Embryology Act in Britain, see: Morgan and Lee (1991); Mulkay (1993, 1994a, 1994b); Squier (1994). For anthropological accounts, see Cannell (1990); Rivière (1985); Shore (1992); Strathern (1992b). For International Reports, see Gunning 1990.

16   For an account of the abortion debate in Britain in the 1980s, see Science and Technology Subgroup (1991).

17   For an account of the conventional genres of popular narrative, and the bases of their appeal, see Radway (1984).

18   Since the period of this study, accounts of 'failed IVF' have become more common. It is a feature of the time period within which I frame this study, however, that such accounts were unavailable.

19   Key figures in the theorisation of ideas of the natural include Escobar (1994); Haraway (1989, 1991); Rabinow (1992); Strathern (1992a, 1992b); Yanagisako and Delaney 1995. For a review of the cultural analysis of science, and the importance of ideas of the natural to this field, see Franklin (1995c).

20   For additional discussion of 'reflexive modernisation' in relation to ideas of the environment, globalisation and risk, see Beck (1992). For an account of the consumption of nature, see MacNachten and Urry (forthcoming).

3 THE 'OBSTACLE COURSE': THE REPRODUCTIVE WORK OF IVF

1   Material for this part of Chapter 3 was originally presented to the Human Reproduction Study Group of the British Sociological Association in Cambridge in 1989. The contributions of members of that group to this and other sections of the thesis are gratefully acknowledged.

2   The term 'treatment' is used throughout these chapters because it is the language used by women themselves. It should be noted, however, that IVF is not a treatment for infertility, and is misleadingly described as such. Even if it is successful, IVF does nothing to alter the condition of infertility.

3 The names used in these chapters are pseudonyms, and identifying information is kept to a minimum throughout. Privacy was of paramount concern to many participants in this study. Even the decision by the clinic to allow my initial letter requesting participation in the study was viewed by many couples who refused to be interviewed, and some who were, as an inappropriate breach of privacy. Much as a more nuanced portrait of individual participants would have enhanced the ethnographic quality of this study, the recording of details about background, religious preference, and even employment was often resisted.

4 This expression of belief is very similar to that discussed by Williams (1988a), in which she considers why women continue to attempt IVF after serial failures. See also Koch (1990).

5 Further sections on coping with failure are included in the subsequent two chapters, where the psychological and emotional consequences of the relativity of success and failure are considered in more depth.

6 For a discussion of the consequences of higher order births, see Botting, et al. (1990); Price (1992).

7 Although this is one of the few direct references to the kinds of media portrayal described earlier, it indicates an awareness of a certain media image of IVF which can be assumed to have also influenced other participants in the study.

8 A 'chemical pregnancy' was the term used to describe positive results of very early tests to determine whether the embryo had implanted. This is a different sort of 'tentative pregnancy' to that described by Rothman (1986) in which a similar element of technological-dependency created an ambivalent feeling towards pregnancy.

9 See, for example, Ann Oakley's classic studies on housework (1974, 1975).

10 The references here to living, eating and drinking IVF not only indicate the extent to which IVF 'takes over', or the extent to which a woman 'becomes her body' (n.b. Martin 1987). They also indicate the extent to which IVF is a 'way of life' that is embodied in more ways than one.

11 This recalls both Martin's arguments about women's self-image in relation to medical representations of their bodies (1987) and also Berger's discussion of the ways in which women see themselves as they are seen by others (1972). For a more complex and positive account of the ways in which women produce objectified images of themselves in the context of IVF, see Cussins (1995, 1997).

12 Modell's account of 'last chance babies' also addresses the issues raised in this passage (1989).

13 The 'professionalisation of fertility management' is also to be found, for example, in the emergence of pre-conceptive care, such as vitamin regimes, which can now comprise part of the process of family planning. Other evidence of this are the advertisements now regularly to be found in women's magazines for ovulation tests which are designed to aid conception. Both Lewin's (1993) and Ginsburg's (1989) accounts of motherhood as an 'achievement' are also relevant to this component of the work of IVF.

14 These more explicit references to self-denial suggest that part of the reason women downplay physical discomfort is related to a wider

phenomenon of feminine self-sacrifice, a trait, which is particularly associated with motherhood. See Jacobus (1990) and Warner (1976: 34–49) for suggestive discussions of self-sacrificial reproductive acts.

15 The way in which IVF changes women's understandings, expectations and identities as a result of the way in which it 'takes over' is an important part of what is meant by the application of the description 'rite of passage' to this procedure. It is in part this change which occurs which it is argued is an undervalued feature of the experience. This is discussed in much greater depth in the next two chapters.

16 For a suggestive discussion of reproductive labour in the form of kinship work, see Leonardo (1987).

4 'IT JUST TAKES OVER': IVF AS AS A 'WAY OF LIFE'

1 The cost of undergoing IVF must be calculated as additional to the cost of the procedure itself, which could in the 1980s range from £850 at the 'budget' end, such as the clinic involved in this study, to £2,500 for in-patient and more up-market services, such as Bourne Hall in Cambridge. Travel, accommodation and time off work are the other major costs incurred. The cost of IVF is higher if the NHS does not supply the necessary drugs for superovulation. At the time of the study, a certain degree of anxiety surrounded this aspect of the programme. Although most GPs were willing to prescribe these drugs on one or two cycles, many were reluctant to absorb the huge costs of these drugs (often around £500 per cycle) indefinitely, and some were outspokenly critical of the technique as a waste of public resources.

2 By 'the context of achieved conception', later referred to as the 'world' of achieved conception, is meant the clinical model of conception derivative of the context of assisted reproduction. In other words, and as is described in more detail below and elsewhere (Franklin 1992a, 1991b), it describes the model of conception as mediated by the discursive and technological apparatus of clinical assistance to procreation.

3 In her early study of amniocentesis (1989), Rayna Rapp uses the term 'moral pioneers' to describe women as they confront the uncertain moral territory presented to them in the context of assisted reproduction. Indeed, there are many senses in which women might be described as 'pioneers' in this context, and might well describe themselves as such, although this is a very American analogy.

4 For literature on the experience of infertility, see in particular Pfeffer and Woollett (1983) and Monach (1993).

5 In relation to the subject of 'life's progression', the interviews replicated very closely the terms of the media accounts. This overlap underscores the central importance of traditional family values to the successful marketing and social acceptance of new forms of reproductive assistance.

6 The use of the language of 'naturalness' to describe fertility is, of course, particularly ironic in the context of achieved conception, where the definitive condition is, rather, artifice.

7 I am here deliberately making reference to the title of Barbara Katz Rothman's book, *The Tentative Pregnancy* (1986), and to her argument that technology renders pregnancy tentative. This idea of technological dependence creating the condition of 'tentativeness' is widely applicable in relation to new reproductive technologies in general, and IVF in particular.

8 This is not to deny that life is fundamentally unpredictable. It is the particular expectation of control expressed here which must be put into perspective. The idea is that some forms of lack of control are more acceptable than others: there are some things 'you just can't help'. There are others where it is seen as necessary to 'try harder' to gain a semblance of control. There are countless moments when people must live with insecurity. What matters here is how reproductive insecurity becomes considered unacceptable and intolerable in relation to normative expectations about children and families.

9 Such comments also demonstrate the extent to which women's sexuality remains defined by their reproductive function. The reference here is not only to impotence (also often linked to sexual identity in men) but to castration (which, in contrast, is not so often associated with infertility in men, as is made evident in expressions such as 'shooting blanks').

10 The emphasis in this description upon 'failed production' directly supports Martin's (1987) argument concerning women's internalisation of dominant medical models of female reproductive capacity as profligate and badly designed. Martin also argues that middle-class women are more likely to internalise such models, due to their greater comparative 'investment' in dominant, normative values. This would, of course, apply precisely to the situation of IVF, which almost exclusively involves a comparatively privileged group.

11 The desire to have children because of the material wealth one has to offer to them instantiates both the enterprise-culture definition of parenthood and the Thatcherite impetus to construct the family as the definitive unit of consumption as noted in Chapter 2 (see also Franklin, Lury and Stacey 1991; McNeil 1991).

12 Judith Lorber's (1989) concept of 'the patriarchal bargain' is also relevant here.

13 This finding confirms that of Crowe's (1989) Australian study of women's motivations in the context of IVF.

14 Several researchers have commented upon the desireability of a study specifically concerned with couples who refuse the option of IVF, and I am often questioned on this point. There are certain logistical difficulties locating a population of 'refusers'. One can speculate that such a group would either have strong values preventing them from pursuing IVF, or would not be as concerned to define their lives according to dominant, normative conventions as is the sample population described here. Such a study would be of particular interest in relation to Martin's empirical finding and consequent hypothesis that degrees of material privilege are correlated to degrees of acceptance of medicalised reproduction (1987).

15 The feeling that 'IVF only makes life more difficult' again expresses the

underside of pain and disappointment to the promise of technological enablement and is discussed in much greater depth in the next chapter.

16 Some of the arguments presented in this section were first presented at the President's Day of the British Association meetings in Swansea in August 1990, organised by Professor Margaret Stacey, and published in an anthology edited by her (Stacey 1992).

17 The 'new probe' referred to is a scanner which is inserted vaginally in order to give a 'better view' of the ovaries. Mixed feelings were expressed about 'the new scanner'. Some, such as this speaker, preferred the increased accuracy of the vaginal probe. Others were less enthusiastic. The necessary manipulation of the probe by the clinician to achieve visual control was a source of both joking and some discomfort.

18 'Learning to see' is perhaps an understatement in the context of interpreting a two-dimensional 'slice' of the lower abdominal interior as shown on a monitor via soundwaves emitted from a probe inserted into the vaginal tract.

19 This conflation is notable, and runs through the entire experience of IVF. The point is that the technology, though described as 'assisting' the reproductive process, actually comes to define it by displacing it. Indeed, technology *becomes* the reproductive process, as is here succinctly evidenced in the dual referents of 'cycles'.

20 Here again, the tantalising promise of technology is so far from its 'deliverables' that it becomes apparent that investment in it is not entirely *about* the deliverables. Again, the investment is about hope: IVF must be understood in part as a 'hope-technology'. Even when women *know it is most likely to fail*, even when they do not even *expect* it to work, the investment is seen to be 'worth it'. One answer to this apparent conundrum is that it is not the expectation it will work which appeals, but the occasion for hope, fantasy, romance, heroism or other, non-'rational', desires to be satisfied which it offers. This phenomenon is much more well-established in the context of surrogacy, and should act as a reminder that reproduction is 'wonderful and mystical' as well as biologically functional (see Ragoné 1994).

21 The ways in which IVF can become an end in itself are explained in part by the 'hope' it offers. Hence, the relationship to the technology becomes a relationship of hope, and about preserving hope. In turn, the technology can 'succeed' in providing this hope, even if it fails to deliver, as it were. It is the balance between IVF 'being worth it for the hope it gives you' and 'just too much' when it fails that must continually be renegotiated.

22 I am indebted to Faye Ginsburg for drawing my attention to the importance of the clinic as a modern liminal space.

23 This example of 'resistance' presents an interesting contrast to Martin's (1987) study. In her account, 'resistance' took a variety of forms, from direct avoidance to 'oppositional consciousness'. The example here is of resistance from within the clinical setting and adds suggestively to the range of resistances available to, and undoubtedly widely practiced by, women in the context of medical management of their bodies (see also Cussins, 1995, 1997).

24 The idea of self-management here, as well as the techniques of visualisation and 'positive-thinking' employed, also evoke the context

of 'alternative medicine'. Whilst in one sense a form of 'resistance', this can also be seen as a capitulation to an individualistic model of health, whereby people are made responsible for their own diseases via their lifestyles. See further in Coward (1988), Stacey (forthcoming).

25 There is, however, a double-edged nature to this valorisation, as it is arguably not just the woman's welfare which is the reason for her 'special' provision, but much less personal concerns, such as providing a competitive service, advancing research goals, procuring 'spare' embryos, increasing the clinic's success rates, and so forth.

26 Many women recounted very disturbing episodes of reproductive illness or malfunction, or both. Two women had nearly died from undiagnosed conditions, and many women's lack of adequate reproductive healthcare (or for that matter, any reproductive healthcare at all) was the suspected, or known, cause of their infertility.

27 Also evident in this statement is the expansion of parenthood effected by the provision of reproductive assistance. Not only penetration, but fertilisation and impregnation are performed by the clinician, who thus acquires what is conventionally understood as the role definitive of fatherhood.

28 Although the quality of care at private clinics was routinely praised, and often contrasted against unpleasant experiences on the NHS, a woman died shortly after this study was completed at the clinic where I conducted this research. The cause was 'ovarian hyperstimulation', a leading cause of fatality on IVF programmes.

29 A direct consequence of Thatcherism was also an increased burden on 'the community' (i.e. women) to 'pick up' some of the slack produced by cuts to the NHS. This also impacted directly the lives of women service providers in the public sector. Hence, while appearing to 'widen' consumer choices, Thatcherism also directly limited many women's lives by adding an increased burden of care and provision, both in the home and through the traditionally female professions of nursing and social work (see McNeil 1991).

30 This again can be understood in terms of all of the things IVF can 'deliver' in addition to a baby. It was sometimes my feeling that women's pursuit of IVF motherhood was like a woman's equivalent to war. Her body *was* 'the front line', and she had the scars to prove her bravery in the pursuit of motherhood. If motherhood is to the establishment of womanhood what warfare is to the establishment of manhood, then this analogy provides a very different picture of the woman lying on the table during aspiration.

31 In addition to being described as 'miracle babies', IVF offspring are also referred to as 'precious babies'. This has a double-referent, both to the cost of IVF and to the fact that these children are seen as especially wanted because of what their parents went through to get them.

32 In the classic romance narrative is required an obstacle to fulfilment, thus producing the requisite tension and anticipation from which much of the pleasure associated with this genre is derived (Radway 1984). Though it may well be that an obstacle to parenthood is not experienced in this way, it may well serve not unrelated functions.

33 Here again it is 'the hope that it offers' which can make IVF

'worthwhile', in so far as the preservation of hope, 'keeping hope alive', can become a goal in itself. In this sense, IVF can be seen as a devotional activity built around faith, faith in a technological 'miracle'. These issues are discussed at greater length in Chapter 8.

34 That women have later regrets is demonstrated by the extract from a radio broadcast discussed in the next chapter, in which one of the women interviewed for this study voices her regrets about the procedure.

35 Concern about the use of in vitro fertilisation has been the subject of considerable feminist debate since the mid-1980s. From specific concerns about the adverse effects of drugs used to super-ovulate women (Klein and Rowland 1988, 1989), to more general critiques of the patriarchal nature of high-technology reproductive intervention (Rothman 1989, Corea 1985, Spallone 1989), feminist writings on the subject of new reproductive technologies have emerged as a major area of late twentieth-century feminist scholarship. See also Birke, *et al.*, 1990; McNeil, *et al.*, 1990; O'Brien 1981; and Stanworth 1987.

5 'HAVING TO TRY' AND 'HAVING TO CHOOSE': HOW IVF 'MAKES SENSE'

1 Such a description also contrasts rather starkly with the image of women as 'passive' in relation to reproductive technology.

2 This situation of unsatisfactory 'choices' corresponds to Rothman's (1984) similar descriptions of 'choices' in the context of amniocentesis.

3 Although menopause is often seen as a 'natural boundary' to a woman's fertility, there are already cases of post-menopausal women giving birth via IVF. Hence, even this potential point of 'finality' to a woman's fertility is now provisional in the context of assisted reproduction. Indeed, the period of ovulation induction is also referred to as 'artificial menopause' in that the pituitary gland is blocked and an artificial 'cycle' produced by hormonal injections.

4 Here again, IVF can be seen as a 'hope technology'.

5 In such contradictory statements is evident the difficulty of assuming that even women's own descriptions of their experience represent a complete account. As experience is itself composed of contradictory components, there are clearly multiple and simultaneously conflicting 'truths' to the 'reality' of experience.

6 In their account of the development of IVF, Edwards and Steptoe (1980) affirm their mutual interest in the research benefits of this technique over and above its potential usefulness for infertility treatment. For further discussion, see Spallone (1989).

7 In this description is also evident the inappropriateness of the term 'desperate', so ubiquitously used to describe infertile couples.

8 The definition of 'mother' in the Human Fertilisation and Embryology Act of 1990 is similarly defined in technological terms. Clause 27 states that a mother is to be defined as 'the woman who is carrying or has carried a child as a result of *the placing in her* of an embryo or of sperm and eggs' (emphasis added).

9 Again, it is determination rather than 'desperateness' which could be

said to characterise women undergoing IVF. This is not only a more flattering description, but one that correctly identifies her active desires in relation to treatment as opposed to an image of near pathological need.

10 Ethnographic work on surrogacy in the US by anthropologist Helena Ragoné suggests an 'ends over means' rationale by which the unconventional nature of procreation in the context of emergent reproductive options is mitigated by a strong emphasis on the outcome, or end result. The point is to end up with a proper nuclear family, in which case it does not really matter how you 'achieved' it, would be the argument (Ragoné, personal communication, see also 1994).

11 The idea of 'giving nature a helping hand', for example, is described earlier in the analysis of IVF pamphlets. For an analysis of the Organon video 'When Nature Fails', see Burfoot (1990: 70–1).

12 The reference is to two films shown on British television in March of 1988 entitled 'The Agony and the Ecstasy' and 'The World of the Unborn'. This was one of the few references to media sources mentioned in the interviews. For an analysis of these films, see Franklin (1991b).

13 This comment also happens neatly to encapsulate the 'problem' of the 'virgin birth' debates!

14 Martin's (1987) analysis of scientific constructions of female reproductive capacity as 'badly designed' is clearly relevant in this context.

15 Nature, defined mechanistically, thus becomes a metaphor for scientific intervention, which is defined naturalistically. In such cross-borrowing is rendered somewhat dubious the distinction between these otherwise seemingly opposing categories.

16 This possibility for vicarious participation in 'something greater than the individual' has many dimensions, including the celebrity attached to IVF, the potential to 'embody progress' as well as a 'miracle baby', the heroism of IVF and also a certain altruism which can be seen on numerous occasions. Undertaking IVF can thus be seen as a choice formulated in relation not only to an individual's, or a couple's, reproductive future, but for 'the future' in several other senses, most notably in terms of scientific progress. IVF, even when it fails, can be seen in this way as contributing to the welfare of the next generation, both in literally bearing it and in contributing to its welfare more indirectly.

17 Neither these chapters nor this book cover the extensive feminist debate of new reproductive technologies. For a useful introduction, see Arditti (1984); Stanworth (1987); Steinberg and Spallone (1988); McNeil (1990); Stacey (1992). For representative debate, see Rapp (1988) and for a summary, see Franklin (1992b).

6 THE EMBODIMENT OF PROGRESS

1 I have elsewhere written at greater length on the parliamentary debate of the Human Fertilisation and Embryology Act, and on the question of postmodern, or cyborg, kinship (Franklin 1993a). Here, I offer selective exemplification which repeats somewhat that longer argument, however in relation to a different frame of reference.

2 For more detailed historical discussion of the overlap between notions of mental and procreative conception, see Stafford (1991), Laqueur (1990) and Battersby (1994). I have elsewhere developed this argument specifically in relation to scientific epistemology (Franklin 1995d).

3 The woman in question miscarried shortly after her experience was described in Parliament.

4 It should be noted, however, that the devotion of scientists is not always towards the same end as that of the devotional would-be mother. A revealing portrait of the fortuitous dovetailing between IVF as an infertility treatment and its usefulness as a research technique is provided in Edwards and Steptoe's account of the development of IVF, entitled *A Matter of Life* (1980). See also Edwards 1989.

5 The *Report of the Committee on the Ethics of Gene Therapy* was published in January of 1992 (Cm 1788). It states there are no new ethical issues arising out of gene therapy, which it compares to organ transplants. Such a position illustrates the enormous faith in the capacity to 'assist' genealogy characteristic of British public and scientific debate in this period. A very useful documentation of the history of assistance to genealogy in the form of modern English breeding practices is provided by Russell (1986). See also Ritvo (1987).

6 See Jacobus (1990) and Warner (1976) for a discussion of religious imagery that is highly relevant to the context of IVF.

7 For an account of the ubiquity of religious imagery in the context of new genetic technologies, see Nelkin and Lindee's account of 'sacred DNA' (1995: 38–57). See also Duden (1993b) and Haraway (forthcoming) on the sacralisation of life itself. I have written elsewhere on the history of western definitions of 'life' (1995b), the 'fetishism' of the gene (1988), the new genetic essentialism (1993b) and emergent definitions of 'life itself' (1993c, 1995a, 1995b).

8 In arguing that the continuity of scientific knowledge, as well as the normative ideals of conjugality and procreativity, are conjoined, celebrated and embodied through the 'miracle baby', I would add that it is no coincidence such babies are almost exclusively white, at least in Britain. Since no statistics are available on the racial composition of the test-tube baby population, my basis for this claim is anecdotal. However, there is a very notable contrast between the fervent pronatalism expressed in the context of IVF, and the demonisation of single, working-class, inner-city, and especially immigrant mothers expressed in other public debates at the time of this study.

9 This argument can be equally powerfully made in relation to information technologies, as has so powerfully been demonstrated by Stefan Helmreich's revealing fieldwork among artifical life scientists at the Santa Fe Institute for the Study of Complexity (1995, 1997). Demonstrating how such scientists not only claim their virtual creations to be 'alive', but to be their informatic progeny, Helmreich neatly illustrates the collapse of authorship, invention and scientific discovery with paternity or genius.

10 The increasing recognition of 'science' as a cultural system deprives the 'biological facts of human reproduction' of their unmediated scientific authority, in the same way that new indeterminacies about the biogenetic

events of conception trouble their more concrete or literal self-evidentness. These 'facts' are thus doubly deprived of their former
obviousness – both in terms of their status as 'scientific' and in terms
of their 'actual' workings.

11 In using this definition of postmodernism, I am relying in part on the
definitions provided by both Beck (1992) and Lyotard (1984).

12 The 'medicalisation of consanguinity' is a term which derives from a co-
authored *Report* to the European Commission Human Genome Analysis
Programme under its Social, Legal and Ethical Implications scheme
(Franklin and Strathern 1993).

Bibliography

Abercrombie, Nicholas and Keat, Russell (eds) (1991) *Enterprise Culture*, London: Routledge.

Arditti, Rita, Klein, Renate Duelli and Minden, Shelley (1984) *Tube Women: What Future For Motherhood?* London: Pandora Press.

Aries, P. (1962) *Centuries of Childhood* (trans. R. Baldick), London: Cape.

Austen, L. (1934) 'Procreation among the Trobriand islanders', *Oceania* 5: 102–13.

Bachofen, J.J. (1861)[1967] *Das mutterrecht*, printed in English as *Myth, Religion and Mother-right* (trans by R. Mannheim), Princeton, NJ: Bolingen Series 84.

Barnes, J.A. (1961) 'Physical and social kinship', *Philosophy of Science* 28: 296–9.

—— (1963) 'Introduction' to *The Family among the Australian Aborigines*, B. Malinowski (rev. edn) New York: Schocken Books.

—— (1964) 'Physical and social facts in anthropology', *Philosophy of Science* 1: 294–7.

—— (1973) 'Genetrix: Genitor: Nature: Culture', in J. Goody, (ed.) *The Character of Kinship*, Cambridge: Cambridge University Press.

Battersby, Christine (1989[1994]) *Gender and Genius: Towards a Feminist Aesthetics*, London: The Women's Press.

Beck, Ulrich (1992) *Risk Society: Towards a New Modernity* (trans. by M. Ritter), London: Sage.

Beer, Gillian (1983) *Darwin's Plots: Evolutionary Narrative in Darwin, George Eliot and Nineteenth Century Fiction*, London: Routledge & Kegan Paul.

Bellina, Joseph and Wilson, Josleen (1986) *The Fertility Handbook: A Positive and Practical Guide*, Harmondsworth: Penguin.

Berger, John (1972) *Ways of Seeing*, Harmondsworth: Penguin.

Biersack, A. (1983) 'Boundblood: Paela "conception" theory interpreted', *Mankind* 14: 2: 85–100.

Birke, Lynda, Himmelweit, Susan and Vines, Gail (1990) *Tomorrow's Child: Reproductive Technologies in the 1990s*, London: Virago Press.

Bloch, M. and Jean, H. (1980) 'Women and the dialectics of nature in C18

French thought', in C. MacCormack and M. Strathern (eds) *Nature, Culture and Gender*, Cambridge: Cambridge University Press.

Botting, Beverley, Macfarlane, Alison and Price, Frances (1990) *Three, Four and More: A Study of Triplet and Higher Order Births*, London: HMSO.

Bouquet, Mary (1993) *Reclaiming English Kinship: Portuguese Refractions of British Kinship Theory*, Manchester: Manchester University Press.

—— (1994) 'Family trees and their affinities', paper prepared for the international symposium, *What's Blood Got To Do With It? Kinship Reconsidered*, Anthropology Board, University of California, Santa Cruz, 29 April – 1 May published in the Journal of the Royal Anthropological Institute 2:1: 43–67, March 1996).

—— (1995a) 'Strangers in Paradise: an encounter with Fossil Man at the Dutch National Museum of Natural History' in *Science as Culture*.

—— (1995b) 'Displaying Knowledge: the trees of Haeckel. Dubois, Jesse and Rivers at the *Pithecanthropus* centennial exhibition' in M. Strathern, (ed.) *Shifting Contexts*, London: Routledge pp. 31–56.

Brown, Lesley, and Brown, John with Freeman, Sue (1979) *Our Miracle Called Louise*, London: Paddington Press.

Burfoot, Annette (1990) 'The normalisation of a new reproductive technology', in M. McNeil, I. Varcoe and S. Yearley (eds.) *The New Reproductive Technologies*, London: Macmillan, pp. 58–74.

Burridge, K. O. L. (1968) 'Virgin Birth' (correspondence), *Man* 3: 651–6.

Butler, Judith (1990) *Gender Trouble: Feminism and the Subversion of Identity*, New York: Routledge.

Cannell, Fenella (1990) 'Concepts of parenthood: the Warnock Report, the Gillick Debate, and modern myths', *American Ethnologist* 17: 4: 667–86.

Chodrorow, N. (1974) 'Family Structure and Feminine Personality', in M.Z. Rosaldo and L. Lamphere (eds.) *Woman, Culture and Society*, Stanford: Stanford University Press, pp. 43–66.

Cloke, Paul (ed.) (1992) *Policy and Change in Thatcher's Britain*, Oxford: Pergamon Press.

—— Collier, J. and Yanagisako, S. (eds.) (1987a) *Gender and Kinship Theory: Essays Toward a Unified Analysis*, Stanford: Stanford University Press.

—— (1987b) 'Introduction' in J. Collier and S. Yanagisako (eds.) *Gender and Kinship: Essays Toward a Unified Analysis*, Stanford: Stanford University Press, pp. 1–13.

Collier, Jane, Rosaldo, Michelle and Yanagisako, Sylvia (1982) 'Is there a family, new anthropological views', in B. Thorne and M. Yalom (eds.) *Rethinking the Family: Some Feminist Questions*, New York: Longman, pp. 25–39.

Concise Oxford Dictionary (1990) (8th edn), Oxford: Oxford University Press.

Corea, Gena (1985) *The Mother-Machine: Reproductive Technologies from Artificial Insemination to Artificial Wombs*, New York: Harper & Row.

Coward, Rosalind (1983) *Patriarchal Precedents: Sexuality and Social Relations*, London: Routledge & Kegan Paul.

—— (1988) *The Whole Truth*, London: Pluto.

Crowe, Christine (1985) '"Women want it"; in vitro fertilisation and women's motivations for participation', *Women's Studies International Forum* 8: 547–52.

Cunningham, Anne (1988) 'Test-tube boy for thrilled parents', *Daily News*, 29 March: 1.

Cussins, Charis (1995) 'Ontological choreography: agency for women patients in an infertility clinic', forthcoming in Social Studies of Science, 1996.

—— (1997) 'Cycles of conceivability: the construction of the Normal Woman in an infertility clinic', in S. Franklin, S. and H. Ragonè (eds) *Reproducing Reproduction*, Philadelphia: University of Pennsylvania Press.

Davis-Floyd, R. (1992) *Birth as an American Rite of Passage*, Berkeley: University of California Press.

Davis-Floyd, R. and Sargent, L (eds.) (1996), *Childbirth and Authoritative Knowledge: Cross-cultural perspectives*, Berkeley: University of California Press.

Dawkins, Richard (1976) *The Selfish Gene*, Oxford, Oxford University Press.

—— (1986) *The Blind Watchmaker; Why the Evidence of Evolution Reveals a Universe Without Design*, New York: Harper & Row.

De Beauvoir, Simone (1974) *The Second Sex* (trans. by H. M. Parshley), New York: Knopf (1949, Librarie Gallimard).

Delaney, Carol (1986) 'The meaning of paternity and the Virgin Birth debate', *Man* 21(3): 494–513.

—— (1991) *The Seed and the Soil: Gender and Cosmology in Turkish Village Society*, Berkeley: University of California Press.

Department of Health and Social Security (1986) *Legislation on Human Infertility Services and Embryo Research: A Consultation Paper*, London: HMSO (Cm 46).

—— (1987) *Human Fertilisation and Embryology: A Framework for Legislation*, London: HMSO (Cm 259).

Derret, J. M. Duncan (1971) 'Virgin Birth in the Gospels', *Man* 6: 289–93.

Dixon, R. M. W. (1968) 'Virgin Birth' (correspondence), *Man* 3: 651–6.

Donzelot, J. (1980) *The Policing of Families: Welfare Versus the State*, London: Hutchinson (originally published in French 1977).

Douglas, Mary (1969) 'Virgin Birth', *Man* 4: 133–4.

Duden, Barbara (1993a) *The Public Fetus* (extracted in *Science as Culture* 17: 562–600.

—— (1993b) *Disembodying Women: Perspectives on Pregnancy and the Unborn* (trans. by Lee Hoinacki), Cambridge, MA: Harvard University Press.

Dunstan, Gordon (ed.) (1990) *The Human Embryo: Aristotle and the Arabic and European Traditions*, Exeter: University of Exeter Press.

Dunstan, Gordon and Seller, Mary (eds.) (1988) *The Status of the Human Embryo: Perspectives from Moral Tradition*, London: King Edward's Hospital Fund for London.

Edwards, Jeanette, Franklin, Sarah, Hirsch, Eric, Price, Frances and Strathern, Marilyn (1993) *Technologies of Procreation: Kinship in the Age of Assisted Conception*, Manchester: Manchester University Press.

Edwards, Robert (1989) *Life Before Birth: Reflections on the Embryo Debate*, London: Hutchinson.

Edwards, Robert and Steptoe, Patrick (1980) *A Matter of Life*, London: Hutchinson.

Engels, Frederick (1884)[1972] *On the Origins of the Family, Private Property and the State*, New York: International Publishers.

Faderman, L. (1981) *Surpassing the Love of Men: Romantic Friendship and Love Between Women from the Renaissance to the Present*, London: Junction Books.

Fee, Elizabeth (1973) 'The sexual politics of Victorian social anthropology', *Feminist Studies* 2: 23–40.

Filmer, Robert (1630) *Patriarchia*.

Finch, Janet (1989) *Family Obligations and Social Change*, Cambridge: Polity Press.

Firth, R. (ed.) (1957) *Man and Culture: An Evaluation of the Work of Bronislaw Malinowski*, London: Routledge & Kegan Paul.

Fishel, S. and Symonds, E. M. (eds) (1986) *In Vitro Fertilisation: Past, Present, Future*, Oxford: IRL Press.

Ford, Norman (1988) *When Did I Begin?: Conception of the Human Individual in History, Philosophy and Science*, Cambridge: Cambridge University Press.

Fortes, M. (1957) 'Malinowski and the study of kinship', in R. Firth (ed.) *Man and Culture: An Evaluation of the Work of Bronislaw Malinowski*, London: Routledge & Kegan Paul.

—— (1969) *Kinship and the Social Order*, Chicago: Aldine.

Foucault, Michel (1973) *The Order of Things: An Archaeology of the Human Sciences*, New York: Vintage Books.

—— (1976) *The History of Sexuality: Volume One* (trans. by Robert Hurley), Harmondsworth: Penguin Books.

—— (1980) *Herculine Barbin* (trans. by Richard McDougall), Brighton: Harvester Press.

Fox, R. (1967) *Kinship and Marriage: An Anthropological Perspective*, Cambridge: Cambridge University Press.

Franklin, Sarah (1988) 'Lifestory: the gene as fetish object on TV', *Science as Culture* 3, 92–100.

—— (1990a) 'Deconstructing "desperateness": the social construction of infertility in popular representations of new reproductive technologies', in M. McNeil, I. Varcoe and S. Yearley, (eds) *The New Reproductive Technologies*, London: Macmillan, pp. 200–29.

—— (1990b) 'Redefining reproductive choice: the changing landscape of reproductive politics in the context of the new reproductive technologies', paper presented at the London School of Economics.

—— (1991a) 'Fetal fascinations: new dimensions to the medical-scientific construction of fetal personhood', in S. Franklin, C. Lury and J. Stacey (eds) *Off-Centre: Feminism and Cultural Studies*, London: Harper Collins, pp. 190–206.

—— (1991b) 'Postmodern procreation', paper presented at Symposium 113 of the Wenner-Gren Foundation for Anthropological Research, Terrosopolis, Brazil, reprinted in *Science as Culture*, 17: 522–621. F.D. Ginsburg and R. Rapp (eds) *Conceiving the New World Order: The Global Politics of Reproduction*, Berkeley: University of California Press, 1995 pp. 323–75.

—— (1992a) 'Making sense of misconceptions: anthropological perspectives on unexplained infertility', in M. Stacey (ed.) *Changing Human Reproduction: Social Science Perspectives*, London: Sage, pp. 75–91.

—— (1992b) Contested conceptions: a cultural account of assisted reproduction, Ph.D. diss., Centre for Contemporary Cultural Studies, University of Birmingham.

—— (1993a) 'Making representations: parliamentary debate of the Human Fertilisation and Embryology Bill', in J. Edwards *et al.*, *Technologies of Procreation: Kinship in the Age of Assisted Conception*, Manchester: Manchester University Press, pp. 96–131.

—— (1993b) 'Essentialism, which essentialism? Some implications of reproductive and genetic technoscience', *Journal of Homosexuality* 24, 3/4: 27–40.

—— (1993c) 'Life itself', paper presented at the *Detraditionalisation* conference, Centre for the Study of Cultural Values, Lancaster University, 13 June (forthcoming in S. Franklin, C. Lury and J. Stacey, *Second Nature*).

—— (1995a) 'Romancing the helix: nature and scientific discovery', in Jackie Stacey and Lynne Pearce (eds), *Romance Revisited*, London: Lawrence & Wishart, pp. 63–77.

—— (1995b) 'Life', in W. Reich (ed.) *Encyclopaedia of Bioethics*, 2nd edition, New York: Macmillan.

—— (1995c) 'Science as culture, cultures of science', *Annual Review of Anthropology* 24: 163–84.

—— (1996) 'Making Transparencies: Seeing Through the Science Wars', *Social Text* 46–47: 14, 155.

Franklin, Sarah, Lury, Celia, and Stacey, Jackie (1991a) 'Feminism and cultural studies: pasts, presents and futures', in S. Franklin, C. Lury and J. Stacey Jackie (eds) *Off Centre: Feminism and Cultural Studies*, London: HarperCollins, pp. 1–21.

—— (1991b) 'Feminism, Marxism, Thatcherism', in S. Franklin, C. Lury, and J. Stacey (eds) *Off-Centre: Feminism and Cultural Studies*, London: HarperCollins, pp. 21–49.

—— (1991c) (eds) *Off Centre: Feminism and Cultural Studies*, London: HarperCollins.

Franklin, Sarah and McNeil, Maureen (1988) 'Reproductive futures: recent feminist debate of new reproductive technologies', *Feminist Studies* 14,3: 545–74.

Franklin, Sarah and Strathern, Marilyn (1993) *Kinship and the New Genetic Technologies: An Assessment of Existing Anthropological Knowledge*, Report prepared for the Medical Research Division of the European Commission, Human Genome Analysis Programme EC (Brussels).

Frazer, J.G. (1910) *Totemism and Exogamy*, 4 vols, London.

Fustel de Coulanges, N. D. (1871) *The Ancient City: A Study in the Religion, Laws and Institutions of Ancient Greece and Rome*, Garden City, NJ: Doubleday [1956].

Gilbert, S. and Gruber, S. (1979) *The Mad-Woman in the Attic: the Woman Writer and the nineteenth-century literary imagination*, New Haven: Yale University Press.

Gillison, G (1980) 'Images of nature in Gimi thought', in C. MacCormack and M. Strathern (eds) *Nature, Culture and Gender*, Cambridge: Cambridge University Press.

Ginsburg, Faye (1989) *Contested Lives: The Abortion Debate in an American Community*, Boston: Beacon Press.

Ginsburg, Faye and Rapp, Rayna (eds) (1995) *Conceiving the New World Order: The Global Politics of Reproduction*, Berkeley: University of California Press.

Glass, Robert and Ericsson, Ronald (1982) *Getting Pregnant in the 1980s; New Advances in Infertility Treatment and Sex Pre-Selection*, Harmondsworth: Penguin Books.

Goodale, J.C. (1980) 'Gender, sexuality and marriage: a Kaulong model of nature and culture', in C. MacCormack and M. Strathern (eds) *Nature, Culture and Gender*, Cambridge: Cambridge University Press.

Goody, J. (ed.) (1973) *The Character of Kinship*, Cambridge: Cambridge University Press.

Gunning, Jennifer (1990) *Human IVF, Embryo Research, Fetal Tissue for Research and Treatment, and Abortion: International Information*, London: HMSO.

Hall, Stuart (1988) *The Hard Road to Renewal*, London: Verso.

Haraway, Donna (1976) *Crystals, Fabrics and Fields*, New Haven: Yale University Press.

—— (1989) *Primate Visions: Gender, Race and Nature in the World of Modern Science*, London: Free Association Books (New York, Routledge).

—— (1991) *Simians, Cyborgs and Women: The Reinvention of Nature*, London: Free Association Books (New York, Routledge).

—— (1995) 'Universal donors in a vampire culture: It's all in the family: biological kinship categories in the twentieth-century United States', in W. Cronon (ed.) *Uncommon Ground: Toward Reinventing Nature*, Boston: Norton pp. 321–378.

Harding, Stephen (1988) 'Trends in permissiveness', in R. Jowell, S. Witherspoon and L. Brook (eds.) *British Social Attitudes: the Fifth Report*, London: Gower, pp. 35–52.

Harris, O. (1980) 'The power of signs: gender, culture and the wild in the Bolivian Andes', in C. MacCormack and M. Strathern (eds) *Nature, Culture and Gender*, Cambridge: Cambridge University Press.

Hartland, E. S. (1909) *Primitive Paternity*, 4 vols, London.

Hartmann, Betsy (1987) *Reproductive Rights and Wrongs*, New York: Harper & Row.

Hastrup, K. (1974) 'The sexual boundary–purity: heterosexuality and virginity', *Journal of the Anthropological Society of Oxford* 5.

—— (1978) 'The semantics of biology: virginity', in S. Ardener (ed.) *Defining Females*, London: Croom Helm.

Haüser-Schäublin, Brigitta (1989) 'The fallacy of 'real' and 'pseudo' procreation', *Zeitschrift für Ethnologie* 114: 179–94.

Hayden, Cori (1995) 'Gender, genetics and generation: reformulating biology in lesbian kinship' *Cultural Anthropology*.

—— (1997) 'Biodiversity, salvage and the commodification of genetic resources', in S. Franklin and H. Ragone (eds) *Reproducing Reproduction*, Philadelphia: University of Pennsylvania Press.

Helmreich, Stefan (1995) 'Anthropology inside and outside the looking-glass worlds of artifical life', PhD.diss., Department of Anthropology, Stanford University.

Helmreich, Stephen (1995) (1997) 'Replicating reproduction in artificial life: or, the essence of life in the age of virtual electronic reproduction', in S. Franklin and H. Ragone (eds) *Reproducing Reproduction*, Philadelphia: University of Pennsylvania Press.

Herschberger, Ruth (1970) *Adam's Rib*, New York: Harper & Row (originally 1948).

Hiatt, L. R. (1971) 'Secret pseudo-procreation rites among the Australian Aborigines', in L.R. Hiatt and Jayawardina (eds) *Anthropology in Oceania: Essays Presented to Ian Hogbin*, Sydney: Angus and Robertson.

Holmes, Helen and Tymstra, Tjeerd (1987) 'In vitro fertilisation in the Netherlands: experiences and opinions of Dutch women', *Journal of In Vitro Fertilisation and Embryo Transfer* 4, 2: 116–23.

Homans, Hilary (ed.) (1986) *The Sexual Politics of Reproduction*, Aldershot: Gower.

Hopkins, Ellen (1992) 'Tales from the baby factory', *New York Times Sunday Magazine*, 15 March, pp. 40–1, 79–84, 90.

Hubbard, R. and Wald, E. (1993) *Exploding the Gene Myth*, Boston: Beacon Press

Interim Licensing Authority (1989) *IVF Research in the UK: A Report on Research Licensed by the Interim Licensing Authority (ILA) for Human In Vitro Fertilisation and Embryology 1985–9*, London: Interim Licensing Authority.

—— (1990) *The Fifth Report of the Interim Licensing Authority for Human In Vitro Fertilisation and Embryology*, London: Interim Licensing Authority.

—— (1991) *The Sixth Report of the Interim Licensing Authority for Human In Vitro Fertilisation and Embryology*, London: Interim Licensing Authority.

Inhorn, Marcia (1993) *Quest for Conception*, Philadelphia: University of Pennsylvania Press.

Jacobus, Mary (1990) 'In parenthesis: immaculate conceptions and feminine desire', in M. Jacobus, E.F. Keller and S. Shuttleworth (eds) (1990) *Body/Politics: Women and the Discourses of Science*, New York: Routledge, pp. 11–28.

Jacobus, Mary, Keller, Evelyn Fox and Shuttleworth, Sally (eds) (1990) *Body/Politics: Women and the Discourses of Science*, New York: Routledge.

Jessop, Bob, Bonnett, Kevin, Bromley, Simon and Ling, Tom (1988) *Thatcherism*, London: Polity Press.

Jones, E. (1925) 'Mother-right and the sexual ignorance of savages', *International Journal of Psychoanalysis* 6: 109–30.

Jordanova, Ludmilla (1980) 'Natural facts: a historical perspective on science and sexuality', in C. MacCormack and M. Strathern (eds) *Nature, Culture and Gender*, Cambridge: Cambridge University Press, pp. 42–70.

—— (ed.) (1986) *Languages of Nature: Critical Essays on Science and Literature*, London: Free Association Books.

—— (1989) *Sexual Visions: Images of gender in science and medicine between the eighteenth and nineteenth centuries*, London: Routledge.

Jorgensen, D. (ed) (1983) 'Concepts of conception: procreation ideologies in Papua New Guinea', (Special Issue of *Mankind* 14: 1, Sydney Anthropological Society of New South Wales).

Jowell, Roger, Witherspoon, Sharon and Brook, Lindsay (eds) (1988) *British Social Attitudes: The 5th Report*, Aldershot: Gower.

Kayberry, P. (1968) 'Virgin Birth' (correspondence), *Man* 3: 311–12.

Klein, Renate (ed.) (1989) *Infertility: Women Speak Out About Their Experiences of Reproductive Medicine*, London: Pandora Press.

Klein, Renate and Rowland, Robin (1989) 'Women as test-sites for fertility drugs: clomiphene citrate and hormonal cocktails', *Reproductive and Genetic Engineering* 1,3: 219–37.

Koch, Lene (1990) 'IVF: an irrational choice?', *Reproductive and Genetic Engineering* 3: 225–32.

Laqueur, Thomas (1986) 'Female orgasm, generation, and the politics of reproductive biology', *Representations* 14, 1: 1–82.

—— 1990 *Making Sex: Body and Gender from the Greeks to Freud*, Cambridge, MA: Harvard University Press.

Lasker, Judith and Borg, Susan (1989) *In Search of Parenthood: Coping With Infertility and High Tech Conception*, London: Pandora (US edition, 1987).

Leach, E. R. (1957) 'The epistemological background to Malinowski's empiricism', in R. Firth(ed.) *Man and Culture: An Evaluation of the Work of Bronislaw Malinowski*, London: Routledge & Kegan Paul.

—— (1967) 'Virgin Birth', *Proceedings of the Royal Anthropological Institute* 39–49. (Reprinted in E. Leach *The Structural Study of Myth*, London: Jonathan Cape, 1969).

—— (1968a) 'Virgin Birth' (correspondence), *Man* 3: 128.

—— (1968b) 'Virgin Birth' (correspondence), *Man* 3: 651–6.

Leacock, E. (1981) *Myths of Male Dominance*, New York: Monthly Review Press.

Lee, D. (1940) 'A primitive system of values', *Philosophy of Science* 7: 355–78.

Leonardo, Micaela di (1987) 'The female world of cards and holidays: women, families and the work of kinship', *Signs* 12, 3: 440–53.

Lewin, Ellen (1993) *Lesbian Mothers: Gender and Power in American Culture*, Berkeley: University of California Press.

Lorber, Judith (1987) 'In vitro fertilisation and gender politics', *Women and Health* 13: 117–33.

—— (1988) revised version of above in Elaine Baruch, Amadeo. F. D'Adamo, and Joni Seager (eds) *Embryos, Ethics and Women's Rights: Exploring the New Reproductive Technologies*, New York: Harrington Park Press, pp. 117–26.

—— (1989) 'Choice, gift or patriarchal bargain?: women's consent to in vitro fertilisation in male infertility', *Hypatia* 4, 3: 23–34.

Lyotard, Jean-François (1984) *The Postmodern Condition: A Report on*

Knowledge (trans. by Geoff Bennington and Brian Massumi), Minneapolis: University of Minnesota Press.

McClennan, J. F. (1865) *Primitive Marriage: An Inquiry into the Origin of the Form of Capture in Marriage Ceremonies*, Chicago: University of Chicago Press (P. Riviere, ed., 1970).

—— (1886–7) *Studies in Ancient History*, London: Quant.

MacCormack, C. P. and Strathern, M. (1980) *Nature, Culture and Gender*, Cambridge: Cambridge University Press.

McNeil, Maureen (1987) *Under the Banner of Science: Eracmus Darwin and His Age*, Manchester: Manchester University Press. (1991a) 'Putting the Alton Bill in context', in S. Franklin, C. Lury and J. Stacey (eds) *Off-Centre: Feminism and Cultural Studies*, London: HarperCollins, pp. 149–59.

—— (1991b) 'Making and not making the difference: the gender politics of Thatcherism', in S. Franklin, C. Lury and J. Stacey (eds) *Off-Centre: Feminism and Cultural Studies*, London: HarperCollins, pp. 221–41.

McNeil, Maureen and Franklin, Sarah (1991) 'Science and technology: questions for cultural studies', in S. Franklin, C. Lury and J. Stacey (eds) *Off-Centre: Feminism and Cultural Studies*, London: HarperCollins, pp. 129–46.

—— (1993) 'Editorial: procreation stories', *Science as Culture* 17: 477–82.

McNeil, Maureen, Varcoe, Ian, and Yearley, Steven (eds) (1990) *The New Reproductive Technologies*, London: Macmillan.

Maine, H. S. (1861) *Ancient Law: Its Connection with the Early History of Society, and its Relation to Modern Ideas*, Tucson, Arizona: University of Arizona Press [1986].

Malinowski, B. (1913) *The Family among Australian Aborigines*, London: University of London Press.

—— (1916) '*Baloma*: spirits of the dead in the Trobriand islands', *Journal of the Royal Anthropological Institute* 46: 354–430.

—— (1923) 'The psychology of sex and the foundations of kinship in primitive societies', *Psyche* Vol IV (October): 98–128.

—— (1927a) *Sex and Repression in Savage Society*, New York: Meridian.

—— (1927b) *The Father in Primitive Psychology*, New York: W. W. Norton.

—— (1929) *The Sexual Life of Savages*, New York: Harcourt, Brace & World, Inc.

—— (1962) 'Parenthood: the basis of social structure', in *Sex, Culture and Myth*, New York: Harcourt, Brace & World, Inc (originally appeared in V.F. Calverton (ed.) *The New Generation: The Intimate Problems of Parents and Children*, London: Allen & Unwin, 1930).

—— (1937) 'Foreword' to M.F. Ashley-Montagu *Coming Into Being Among the Australian Aborigines: A Study of the Procreative Beliefs of the Native Tribes of Australia*, London: George Routledge & Sons, pp. xix–xxxv.

Marcus, George E. (1995) 'Ethnography in/of the world system: the emergence of multi-sited ethnography, *Annual Review of Anthropology* 24: 95–117.

Martin, Emily (1987) *The Woman in the Body: A Cultural Analysis of Reproduction*, Boston: Beacon Press.

—— (1991) 'The Egg and the Sperm', *Signs* 16, 3: 485–501.

Mathieu, N. C. (1978a) 'Man-culture and woman-nature', *Women's Studies International Quarterly* 1: 55–65.

Matthews, I. and Jones, G. (1987) 'Our gorgeous tiny wonders', *Daily News*, 3 December.

Modell, Judith (1986) 'In search: the purported biological basis of parenthood', *American Ethnologist* 13: 646–61.

—— (1989) 'Last chance babies: interpretations of parenthood in an IVF program', *Medical Anthropology Quarterly* 3: 124–38.

Monach, J. (1993) *Childless: No Choice: the Experience of Involuntary Childlessness*, London: Routledge.

Montagu, Ashley (1937) *Coming into Being among Australian Aborigines: A Study of the Procreative Beliefs of the Native Tribes of Australia*, London: George Routledge Sons, Inc. (2nd revised edn, 1974, London: Routledge & Kegan Paul.

—— (1949) 'Embryological beliefs of primitive peoples', *Ciba Symposia* 10: 994–1008.

Montague, S. (1971) 'Trobriand kinship and the Virgin Birth controversy', *Man* 6: 353–68.

—— (1973) 'Copulation in Kaduwaga' (correspondence), *Man* 8: 304–5.

Morgan, Derek and Lee, Robert (eds) (1989) *Birthrights: Law and Ethics at the Beginnings of Life*, London: Routledge.

—— (1991) *Human Fertilisation and Embryology Act 1990: Abortion and Embryo Research, the New Law*, London: Blackstone Press.

Morgan, L. H. (1871) *Systems of Consanguinity and Affinity in the Human Family*, Smithsonian Contributions to Knowledge.

Mosko, Mark (1983) 'Conception, De-Conception and Social Structure in Bush Mekeo culture', *Mankind*: 14: 1: 24–32.

Mountford, C. P. (1981) *Aboriginal Conception Beliefs*, Melbourne: Hyland House.

Mulkay (1993) 'Rhetorics of hope and fear in the great embryo debate', *Social Studies of Science* 23: 721–42.

—— (1994a) 'Changing minds about embryo research', *Public Understanding of Science* 3: 195–213.

—— (1994b) 'Embryos in the news', *Public Understanding of Science* 3: 33–51.

Nader, L. (ed.) (1996) *Naked Science: Anthropological Inquiry into Boundaries, Power and Knowledge*, New York: Routledge.

Needham, J. (1975) *A History of Embryology*, New York: Arno.

Nelkin, Dorothy and Lindee, Susan (1995) *The DNA Mystique: The Gene as Cultural Icon*, New York: W. H. Freeman.

Newbold, Anne (1987) 'Joy for baby hope couples', *Daily News* 19 March: 1.

Oakley, Ann (1974) *Housewife*, Harmondsworth: Penguin Books.

—— (1975) *The Sociology of Housework*, London: Martin Robertson.

O'Brien, Mary (1981) *The Politics of Reproduction*, Boston: Routledge & Kegan Paul.

Ortner, Sherry (1974) 'Is Female to Nature as Male is to Culture', in M. Rosaldo and L. Lamphere (eds) *Culture and Society*, Stanford, CA: Stanford University Press, pp. 67–96.

Parsons, A. (1964) 'Is the Oedipus complex universal? The Jones-Malinowski debate revisited and a South Italian "nuclear complex"', *The Psychoanalytic Study of Society*, 3: 278–328.

Pearson, Maggie (1992) 'Health', in P. Cloke (ed.) *Policy and Change in Thatcher's Britain*, Oxford: Pergamon Press, pp. 215–46.

Perloe, Mark and Christie, Linda Gail (1986) *Miracle Babies and Other Happy Endings: How Modern Medical Advances Can Help Couples Conceive*, New York: Rawson Associates.

Petchesky, Rosalind Pollack (1987) 'Foetal images: the power of visual culture in the politics of reproduction', in M. Stanworth (ed.) *Reproductive Technologies: Gender, Motherhood and Medicine*, London: Polity Press, pp. 81–97.

Pfeffer, Naomi (1987) 'Artificial insemination, *in vitro* fertilisation and the stigma of infertility', in M. Stanworth (ed.) *Reproductive Technologies: Gender, Motherhood and Medicine*, London: Polity Press.

Pfeffer, Naomi and Quick, Allison (1988) *Infertility Services: A Desperate Case*, London: Greater London Association of Community Health Care.

Pfeffer, Naomi and Woollett, Anne (1983) *The Experience of Infertility*, London: Virago.

Poole, F. J. P. (1981) 'Transforming "natural" woman: female ritual leaders and gender ideology among Bimin Kuskusmin', in S. Ortner and H. Whitehead (eds) *Sexual Meanings: The Cultural Construction of Gender and Sexuality*, Cambridge: Cambridge University Press, pp. 116–166.

—— (1984) 'The fecundity of a "procreative model" in the analysis of gender and kinship', *Social Analysis* 16.

Powell, H. A. (1968) 'Virgin Birth' (correspondence), *Man* 3: 651–2.

—— (1969a) 'Genealogy, residence and kinship in Kiriwina', *Man* 4: 177–202.

—— (1969b) 'Territory, hierarchy and kinship in Kiriwina', *Man* 4: 580–604.

Prentice, Thomson (1986) 'Living in limbo, longing for life', *The Times*, 8 April: 13.

—— (1986) 'The test-tube maybe. . . .', *The Times*, 9 April: 10.

Price, Frances (1989) 'Establishing guidelines: regulation and the clinical management of infertility', in D. Morgan and R. Lee (eds) *Birthrights: Law and Ethics at the Beginnings of Life*, London: Routledge.

—— (1992) 'Having triplets, quads or quins: who bears the responsibility?', in M. Stacey (ed.) *Changing Human Reproduction: Social Science Perspectives*, London: Sage, pp. 92–118.

Rabinow, Paul (1992) 'Artificiality and enlightenment', in J. Crary and S. Kwinter (eds) *Incorporations*, New York: Zone Books.

Radway, Janice A. (1984) *Reading the Romance: Women, Patriarchy and Popular Literature*, Chapel Hill and London: University of North Carolina Press.

Ragoné, Helena (1994) *Surrogate Motherhood: Conception in the Heart*, Boulder, Co: Westview.

Rapp, Rayna (1982).

—— (1988) 'A womb of one's own' (book review), *The Women's Review of Books* 5, 7(April): 9–10 (see also reply by P. Spallone, *The Women's Review of Books* 5, 10–11(July): 4.

—— (1989) 'Moral pioneers: women, men and fetuses on a frontier of reproductive technology', in E. Baruch, A. D'Adamo and J. Seager (eds) *Embryos, Ethics and Women's Rights*, New York: Harringdon Park Press, pp. 101–16.

Read, C. (1917) 'No paternity', *Journal of the Royal Anthropological Institute*.

Reiter, R. (ed.) (1975) *Toward an Anthropology of Women*, New York: Monthly Review Press.

Rentoul, A. (1931) 'Physiological paternity and the Trobrianders', *Man* 31: 152–4.

—— (1932) 'Papuans, professors and platitudes', *Man* 32: 274–6.

Ritvo, H. (1987) *'Animal Estate: the English and Other Creatures in the Victorian Age'*, Cambridge: Harvard University Press.

Riviere, Peter (1985) 'Unscrambling parenthood: the Warnock Report', *Anthropology Today* 1, 4: 2–6.

Rivers, W. H. R. (1910) 'The genealogical method of anthropological inquiry' in *Sociological Review* Vol. 3: Manchester and London.

—— (1924) *Social Organisation and Kinship*, London: Athlone Press.

Roheim, G. (1933) 'Women and their life in Central Australia', *Journal of the Royal Anthropological Institute* 63: 207–65.

Rosaldo, Michelle and Lamphere, Louise (eds) (1974a) *Woman, Culture and Society*, Stanford, CA: Stanford University Press.

Rosaldo, M. and Lamphere, L. (1974b) 'Introduction', in M. Rosaldo and L. Lamphere (eds) *Woman, Culture & Society*, Stanford: Stanford University Press.

Rose, Mark (forthcoming) 'From Paternity to Property: the remetaphorization of waiting' in M. Woodmansee and P. Juszi (eds.) *Cultural Agency/ Cultural Authority*, Durham: Duke University Press.

Ross, Andrew (ed.) (1996) 'The science wars', special issue of *Social Text*, 46–47.

Rothman, Barbara Katz (1984) 'The meanings of choice in reproductive technology', in R. Arditti, R.D. Klein and S. Minden (eds) *Test-Tube Women: What Future For Motherhood?*, London: Pandora Press (Routledge & Kegan Paul), pp. 23–34.

—— (1986) *The Tentative Pregnancy: Prenatal Diagnosis and the Future of Motherhood*, New York: Viking.

—— (1989) *Recreating Motherhood: Ideology and Technology in a Patriarchal Society*, New York: W. W. Norton.

Rubin, Gayle (1975) 'The traffic in women: notes on the "political economy" of sex', in R. Reiter (ed.) *Toward an Anthropology of Women*, New York: Monthly Review Press, pp. 157–210.

Ruddick, C. T. (1970) 'Birth narratives in Genesis and Luke', *Novum Testamentum* 12: 438–8.

Russell, N. (1986) 'Like Engend'ring Like: Heredity and Animal Breeding in Early Modern England, Cambridge: Cambridge University Press.

Sacks, K. (1982) *Sisters and Wives: The Past and Future of Sexual Equality*, Illinois: University of Illinois Press.

Sandelowski, Margarete (1993) *With Child in Mind: Studies of the Personal Encounter with Infertility*, Philadelphia: University of Pennsylvania Press.

Savage, Wendy (1986) *A Savage Inquiry*, London: Virago.
Scheffler, H. and Lounsbury, F. (1971) *A Study in Structural Semantics: the Siriono Kinship System*, Englewood Cliffs: Prentice-Hall.
Schiebinger, Londa (1987) 'The history and philosophy of women in science: a review essay', *Signs* 12: 305–32.
—— (1989) *The Mind Has No Sex?: Women in the Origins of Modern Science*, Cambridge, MA: Harvard University Press.
Schneider, David M. (1964) 'The nature of kinship', *Man* 64: 180–1.
—— (1965) 'Kinship and biology', in Ansley J. Coale (ed.) *Aspects of the Analysis of Family Structure*, Princeton: Princeton University Press.
—— (1968a) 'What is kinship all about?', in P. Reining (ed.) *Kinship in the Morgan Centennial Year*, Washington: Anthropological Society of Washington.
—— (1968b) *American Kinship: A Cultural Account*, Englewood Cliffs, NJ: Prentice-Hall.
—— (1968c) 'Virgin Birth' (correspondence), *Man* 3: 126–9.
—— (1984) *A Critique of the Study of Kinship*, Ann Arbor: University of Michigan Press.
Schwimmer, E. (1969) 'Virgin Birth', *Man* 4: 132–3.
Science and Technology Subgroup (1991) 'In the Wake of the Alton Bill: Science, Technology and Reproductive Politics', in S. Franklin, C. Lury, and J. Stacey (eds) *Off-Centre: Feminism and Cultural Studies*, London: HarperCollins, pp. 147–214.
Sharman, G. B. and Pilton, P. (1964) 'The life history and reproduction of the red kangaroo', *Proceedings of the Zoological Society in London* 142: 29–47.
Shore, Chris (1992) 'Virgin births and sterile debates', *Current Anthropology* 33: 3: 295–314.
Sider, K. B. (1967) 'Kinship and culture: affinity and the role of the father in the Trobriands', *Southwest Journal of Anthropology* 23: 90–109.
Singer, Peter and Desole, Daniel E. (1967) 'The Australian Sub incision ceremony reconsidered: vaginal envy or kangaroo biped penis envy?' *American Anthropology* 69: 355–8.
Snowden, Robert and Mitchell, Duncan (1983) *The Artificial Family: A Consideration of Artificial Insemination by Donor*, London: Allen & Unwin.
Spallone, Patricia (1989) *Beyond Conception*, London: Macmillan.
—— (1992) *Generation Games: Genetic Engineering and the Future for Our Lives*, London: The Women's Press.
Spallone, Patricia and Steinberg, Deborah (eds) (1987) *Made to Order: The Myth of Reproductive and Genetic Progress*, London: Pergamon Press.
Spencer, B. and Gillen, F. J. (1899) *The Native Tribes of Central Australia*, London.
Spiro, M. E. (1968) 'Virgin birth, parthenogenesis and physiological paternity: an essay in cultural interpretation', *Man* 3: 242–61.
—— (1972) Reply to Montague (correspondence), *Man* 7: 315.
—— (1984) *Oedipus in the Trobriands*, Chicago: University of Chicago Press.
Squier, Susan Merrill (1994) *Babies in Bottles: Twentieth Century Visions*

of Reproductive Technology, New Brunswick, NJ: Rutgers University Press.

Stacey, J. D. (forthcoming) *Teratologies*, London: Routledge

Stacey, Meg (ed.) (1992) *Changing Human Reproduction: Social Science Perspectives*, London: Sage.

Stafford, Barbara (1991) *Body Criticism: Imaging the Unseen in Enlightenment Art and Medicine*, Cambridge: Mir Press.

Stanworth, Michelle, (ed.) (1987) *Reproductive Technologies: Gender, Motherhood and Medicine*, Cambridge: Polity Press.

Steinberg, Deborah and Spallone, Patricia (eds) (1988) *Made to Order: The Myth of Reproductive and Genetic Progress*, London: Pergamon.

Strathern, Marilyn (1980) 'No nature, no culture', in C.P. MacCormack and M. Strathern (eds) *Nature, Culture and Gender*, Cambridge: Cambridge University Press.

—— (1982) 'Making a difference: connections and disconnections in Highlands kinship systems', paper presented at the Feminism and Kinship conference, Bellagio, Italy, in J. Collier and S. Yanagisako (eds) *Gender and Kinship: Toward a Unified Analysis*, Stanford CA: Stanford University Press, 1987.

—— (1988) *The Gender of the Gift*, Berkeley: University of California Press.

—— (1989) 'Enterprising kinship: consumer choice and the new reproductive technologies', paper presented at the Centre for the Study of Cultural Values, University of Lancaster, in M. Strathern, *Reproducing the Future: Anthropology, Kinship and the New Reproductive Technologies*, Manchester: Manchester University Press, 1992, pp. 31–43.

—— (1990) 'The meaning of assisted kinship', paper presented at the annual Meetings of the British Association for the Advancement of Science, Swansea (M. Stacey 1996), in M. Stacey (ed) *Changing Human Reproduction: Social Science Perspectives*, London: Sage, 1992, pp. 148–169.

—— (1992a) *After Nature: English Kinship in the Late-Twentieth Century*, Cambridge: Cambridge University Press.

—— (1992b) *Reproducing the Future: Anthropology, Kinship and the New Reproductive Technologies*, Manchester: Manchester University Press.

—— (1993) 'A Question of Context' and 'Regulation, Substitution and Possibility' in J. Edwards, *et al.*, *Technologies of Procreation: Kinship in the Age of Assisted Conception*, Manchester: Manchester University Press, pp. 1–19 and 132–161.

—— (1995) *Women in Between: Female Roles in a Male World: Mount Hagen, New Guinea*, London: Rowman and Littlefield (originally published in 1972 by Seminar Press).

Thorne, B. and Yalom, B. (eds.) (1982) *Rethinking the Family: Some Feminist Questions*, New York: Longman.

Tilton, Nan, Tilton, Tod, and Moore, Gaylen (1985) *Making Miracles: In Vitro Fertilisation: A Couple's Triumph Over Infertility*, New York: Doubleday.

Tsing, Lowenhaupt, A. and Yanagisako, Sylvia Junko (1983) 'Feminism and kinship theory', *Current Anthropology* 24: 511–16.

Turner, Victor (1969) *The Ritual Process: Structure and Anti-Structure*, Ithaca, NY: Cornell University Press.

Tylor, E.B. (1871) *Primitive Culture* (2 vols.), London: John Murray.

Van Gennep, Arnold (1906) *The Rites of Passage* (trans. by Monika Vizedom and Gabrielle Caffee), London: Routledge & Kegan Paul.

Voluntary Licensing Authority (1986) *The First Report of the Voluntary Licensing Authority For Human In Vitro Fertilisation and Embryology*, London: Voluntary Licensing Authority.

—— (1987) *The Second Report of the Voluntary Licensing Authority For Human In Vitro Fertilisation and Embryology*, London: Voluntary Licensing Authority.

—— (1988) *The Third Report of the Voluntary Licensing Authority For Human In Vitro Fertilisation and Embryology*, London: Voluntary Licensing Authority.

—— (1989) *The Fourth Report of the Voluntary Licensing Authority for Human In Vitro Fertilisation and Embryology*, London: Voluntary Licensing Authority.

Warner, Marina (1976) *Alone of All Her Sex: The Myth and the Cult of the Virgin Mary*, New York: Knopf.

Warnock, Mary (1985) *A Question of Life*, Oxford: Basil Blackwell.

Weeks, Jeffrey (1981) *Sexuality and its Discontents*, London: Routledge & Kegan Paul.

Weiner, A. (1976) *Women of Value, Men of Renown*, Austin, Texas: University of Texas Press.

—— (1977) 'Trobriand descent: female/male domains', *Ethos* 5: 54–70.

—— (1978) 'The reproductive model in Trobriand society', in J. Specht and P. White *Mankind*, special issue on *Trade and exchange in Oceania and Australia*.

—— (1979) 'Trobriand kinship from another view: the reproductive power of women and men', *Man* 14: 328–348.

—— (1988) *The Trobrianders of Papua New Guinea*, New York: Holt, Rinehart and Winston and (1995) 'Reassessing reproduction in social theory' in F. Ginsburg and R. Rapp (eds) *Conceiving the New World Order: The Global Politics of Reproduction* Berkeley: University of California Press, 407–424.

Weiner, J. (1986) 'Blood and skin: the structural implications of sorcery and procreation beliefs among the Foi', *Ethos* 1–2.

Weston, Kath (1991) *Families we choose: Lesbians, Gays, Kinship*, New York: Columbia University Press.

Westermarck, E. A. (1891)[1921] *The History of Human Marriage, 5th edn*.

Williams, Linda (1988a) '"It's going to work for me": responses to failures of IVF', *Birth* 15, 3: 153–6.

—— (1988b) *Wanting Children Badly: An Exploratory Study of The Parenthood Motivation of Couples Seeking In Vitro Fertilisation*, doctoral dissertation, University of Toronto.

Williams, Peter (1992) 'Housing', in Paul Cloke (ed.) *Policy and Change in Thatcher's Britain*, Oxford: Pergamon Press, pp. 159–98.

Williams, Raymond (1973) *The Country and The City*, Oxford: Oxford University Press.

—— (1981) *Keywords: A Volcabulary of Culture and Society*, London: Fontana.

Wilson, P. J. (1969) 'Virgin Birth' (correspondence), *Man* 4: 286–8.

Winston, Robert (1989) *Getting Pregnant: The Woman's Answer Book*, London: Anaya Publishers.

Yanagisako, S. J. (1985) 'The elementary structure of reproduction in kinship and gender studies', paper presented at the 1985 meeting of the American Anthropological Association, Washington, DC.

Yanagisako, S. J. and Collier, J. (1987) 'Toward a Unified Analysis of Gender and Kinship' in J. Collier and S. Yanagisako. (eds) *Gender and Kinship Theory*, Stanford: Stanford University Press, pp. 14–52.

Yanagisako, S.J. and Delaney, Carol (eds) (1995) *Naturalizing Power: Feminist Cultural Analysis*, New York: Routledge.

Young, R.M. (1985) *Darwin's Metaphor: Nature's Place in Victorian Culture*, Cambridge: Cambridge University Press.

Index